I0390547

To Nurse Means to Nurture
Part Three
Nurses Dealing with Patients with Anxiety Disorders

Brian Evans

Preface

In this book I would like to show how nurses can deal with patients who have anxiety. I have also found comments from college books of nursing and other nursing books I quoted that deal with this area to help me explain to you what I need you to do to help me with my anxiety. The greatest problem I have, plus a lot of other patients have in this area are things like having needle phobia and oversensitivity to pain and fearing others will show them impersonal care because they do not understand their needs or are not willing to meet them. There are also things that autistic people with anxiety fear you will falsely think of them when they say or do odd things. They fear a harsh scolding or punishment because they fear you will consider something to be mischievous in nature they said or did, which from their point of view was innocent in nature because, like in my instance, they are disabled and have the mind of a child. Most of them don't have as many areas of childishness as I do, but they have some areas of childish tendencies. I am childish in a great deal of ways and in other ways I am more mature than most people. Because I was normalized from the Special Ed world into your world and made to look like everyone else it is hard to even tell I have a disability until you are around me a while. If you are one that is quick to judge and condemn it can be too late for the autistic person once you figure out they never meant anything wrong by anything and then both you and them will be very sorry in the end. Nurses need to keep this in mind when dealing with disabled patients. Things are not always what they appear, so don't assume the worst until you see the facts for yourself based on the patient's individuality. Feel out the situation to see how the person thinks and feels before you judge. What may seem mischievous to you may be totally innocent coming from them. In my past experiences, some individuals, mainly in Abilene, Texas and a few at some of the not as understanding hospitals up here would take things I said and make things out of them that were not there.

Brian Evans
2

So, when I start giving my scenario about what you will think or have to say about things I tell you that happened to me as a child, even though they are true, and even though I feel in my heart you already believe me and understand that everything I have to say is true, because of that little flicker of doubt that says, "I don't want to get burned again" I have given examples of what I fear you might think and say about what I have to tell you based on what other judgmental people have said, and then turned the same scenario around to show you where these people are wrong so you can see the truth yourself if you are unable to see the truth. What these doctors, nurses and staff did to me at military hospital and institution may be considered graphic in nature by some individuals. That's why I was afraid you wouldn't believe me. That's the reason I got so defensive is because I was afraid you would think I was lying about it when I was not because I feared you would say, "That kind of thing never happens!" when I told you what happened.

Some of you nice nurses actually know that there are meaner nurses other places that do stuff like this to people and some are even graphic.

Some other nice nurses I've ran into act like they didn't think there was any such thing as a bad nurse because all they ever saw was nice nurses. I wanted to tell you nice nurses that, yes, there are many nurses out there that are nice, but not all nurses are nice.

So, please don't take these negative bias statements I am putting in your mouth that you may think, that probably aren't even things you would think, as suggestions you have something to worry about. Instead see it as my showing you how ignorant people can be because of their false bias about a disabled individual when they aren't completely listening to what their patient is saying. Also, there are many topics I mention I am anxious in this book. There are some of these topics I may talk for several pages about.

There may even be a topic or so that you don't seem to think applies to you and you may feel like, "How long is he going to talk about this anyway? Is the rest of the book about this specific subject?" Let me inform you, I can be very longwinded about things.

I assure you no matter how long I may spend on a certain topic, even the ones you may find unnecessary, I eventually tell about my anxieties over a different topic before I get to the end of the book. I have expressed my emotions in great deal about a lot of stuff I am anxious about to help you understand me. Please do not hold anything against me you may consider inappropriate. Because this is a book about anxiety I wanted to show you the emotions I am feeling over certain things instead of being brief in explaining they are there. Regardless of how silly something sounds and how long it is, I want to be able to show you how I have the emotions of a child so you can see what kinds of things make me anxious, what I'm anxious about, silly or not, and how all this anxiety affects me and what I need you to do to help me deal with these anxieties. So, please be patient with me and please do not punish me for anything you consider to be out of line because I am only trying to show you how certain things make me feel and how they affect me to help you better understand me no matter how silly they may sound.

I actually have my feelings stated about how I want treated in places like the Emergency Room and ICU near the end of the book after I give my long winded scenario about this other stuff I have to say to you. So, please don't miss this part. It is very important you read this.

I also have quotes from College Books of Nursing about how nurses are supposed to treat their patients in the ER in the ICU near the end of the book.

I believe before that I also have comments about what I need to have done for me by everybody everywhere, friends, neighbors, doctors, nurses, techs, and the like after my mother dies.

My mother wants me to be taken care of after she dies and is at the peak of her life expectancy. She will probably only make it another five years, and possibly slightly less. But, I need you to know what these needs are so you know what I need you to do for me when this happens. Please make sure to read this also.

Technically, about the scenario situation, all you would have to do is call my mother and ask her if the things I said these people did to me at the military hospital and the institution is true and she would tell you I am telling you the truth. She was there. She knows exactly what they did and she's known it for decades.

I was just trying to show you how judgmental people can be when they don't believe their patients that they think are different from them and they only listen to half what they are telling them and then come to their own conclusions about what they want to believe happened. It can really be a mess and it can cause a great deal of anxiety and stress and depression for the disabled person you are talking to you're not listening to correctly because of your own bias.

Thankfully, no one at your hospital has pulled this kind of stunt yet. Everyone I have talked to has been very good about taking my word for things.

Some places like to judge before they know the facts, but your place has done really well at taking my word for things and giving me the things I needed for two procedures and in most instances the things I needed in your offices as well. Thank you so much for doing this for me.

Brian Evans

5

When you read all this stuff about the "bias" I fear one of you will think please don't take it to heart. Some of you have only seen me two or three times and others have seen me ten or fifteen times. I'm always worried if someone is not familiar with me and I say or do the least little thing strange because of my disability they will not believe me and show this kind of bias toward me. I am also afraid they will shun me for any oddness they see about me.

Please understand that it is not because of anything you have done that I fear being treated with all this horrible bias but because what others have done in the same regard when they did treat me with all this horrible bias.

This is one of those situations where the last two or three places I went before you guys people would promise to meet certain needs for me and two or three visits later they'd turn the tables on me for no reason and say they couldn't meet them anymore just because they didn't want to meet them because they didn't want to have to treat me like a 5 year old and pamper me all over the place because that made them uncomfortable.

They thought their needs were above the legitimate needs of the patient which I have and they did what they wanted to do and their bias was kicking through where if I did try to state a defense about any past experiences they might try to place the blame on me instead of trying to figure out what really happened and why I really feel the way I do.

Because of this, I feel like I have to go to you a few times to see how you are going to react to me before I can be assured for sure that you are going to follow through for me in continuing to meet my needs and continuing to understand me and comfort and console me in the way I need you to.

Brian Evans

So, if you keep doing this, and you reassure me that you believe me about everything I have to say in this book after you read it and still accept me even after everything you have read here then eventually I can feel at ease with my situation and not have to worry like crazy all the time how you will react to me.

As far as the procedures go, same story.

You've done very well so far.

Once three or four departments have had me go to three or four procedures and shown me they are going to follow through in advocating for me, and once these people they send me to three or four times in a row a piece follow through with meeting all my needs, then I can relax and be reassured that they will meet my needs as well.

If it weren't for people that don't keep their promises I've run into before that do what you want them to do the first time or two and then refuse to follow through ever again after the first couple of times, I wouldn't have this problem.

I'm sorry it has to be like this. I'm trying to trust you to follow through for me, but it is hard to do when my past experiences of people doing this to me has fallen over my head.

That's why I am anxious about all of you guys thinking and doing the things I mentioned in this book, that I really have a feeling you'd never say or do.

I just need continual reassurance.

Some of the things I worry about that are probably far from worrisome that you probably wonder where I got from I talked to an ex-doctor's wife about I was friends with. This lady saw my hospital book on the internet and read it. She may have bought it I'm not sure.

Brian Evans
7

After she did, she said, "I read your book and I've had elephants before, but you have had several big elephants on you that have trampled all over you your entire life, one right after the other. No wonder you have such a problem with doctors and nurses and hospitals. I think you may have Post Traumatic Stress Disorder. You might tell your doctors that the next time you go to it. It might help them understand you better. Maybe they'd give you a little more slack and be nicer to you then. Some of these people just don't understand what you've been through, but this is terrible. You need to tell them this. Maybe then they'll understand you and be more willing to meet your needs."

I hope this helps you understand. I'm sorry if I said anything in this book that offends you guys. I don't think you're anything like these people I'm worried about you acting like in this book. I just have a hard time not getting on the defense because of the way others have acted toward me and because of that little glimmer of doubt, I think, "What if?" and then I really go out on a rampage with it. So, please don't take any of this to heart.

And, please remember, I may think, say, or do some strange things some times or ask strange questions but I have the socialization of a 5 year old and the communication of a 10 year old, and I have the emotional mind of a 5 year old but have the intellect of someone a few years older than that due to memorization of facts in books.

So, if I say something that makes you want to raise your eyebrows and think "What's up with this?" please don't hold this against me and condemn me for it, because whatever it is that makes you feel this way, if I said something that sounds this way to you, it might as well have been a 5 year old that said it or asked it because that's the way I think.

Remember this is a book about anxiety. I want you to be able to see what all I'm worked up about and what you can do to help me relieve my anxiety over these things and not condemn me for it.

Brian Evans
8

Thank you for your compassion and understanding and please continue to treat me with the same comfort and compassion you always have in the same way you always have regardless of how this book makes you feel.

I just want you to understand me as a person and see just how childlike my emotions can be and how traumatizing they can be to me as well no matter how silly they may be. Thanks.

I want you to treat me like I'm your own sweet little boy who means something to you that you want to take care of and show your love and compassion to when you work with me.

If you can still accept me like I am after you read this book and are still willing to meet my needs with the same comfort and compassion in the same you always have then we have it made. Then, I can relax. When you read this book, open your eyes and see who I really am, a child at heart. Please enjoy your read. Thank you.

Your friend,
Brian Gene Evans

To Nurse Means To Nurture Part Three
Nurses Dealing with Patients with Anxiety Disorders

To begin with here are a few quotes I have found that may help nurses understand the effects of anxiety on a patient.

"When action has been taken and the danger is over or the problem resolved, the body relaxes and returns to normal once more."

> Funk and Wagnall's New Illustrated Encyclopedia of Family Health,
> A-B, Marshall Cavendish Limited, Reference Edition, 1988, page 70

On page 69 of Funk and Wagnall's New Illustrated Encyclopedia of Family Health, A,-B, there is a picture of a child being comforted by its mother in its anxiety. The comment attached to this picture says, "A child's anxiety is readily dispelled by the loving reassurance of his mother."

> Funk and Wagnall's New Illustrated Encyclopedia of Family Health,
> A-B, Marshall Cavendish Limited, Reference Edition, 1988, page 69

"Usually we are unable to tolerate anxious feelings for a sustained period of time."

> Basic Nursing, A Psychophysiologic Approach, Sorensen and Luckmann, W.B. Saunders Company 1979, page 121

"The skilled nurse recognizes that illness produces anxious feelings in patients; she also tries to be sensitive to the individual anxieties that patients experience when illness interferes with their unique self-explanations and needs."

> Basic Nursing, A Psychophysiologic Approach, Sorensen and Luckmann, W.B. Saunders Company 1979, page 122

"As a patient's level of anxiety increases he will become increasingly unable to understand clearly what is happening to him and what is expected of him. Thus, if a patient's level of anxiety is excessively high it will interfere with effective patient teaching. Because the extremely anxious person easily misunderstands what is said to him communication with him should be clear and directions brief. Repeating statements is frequently helpful, as an anxious person tend to forget easily. Nonverbal motions may aid in clarifying communication at such times. The anxious person needs an opportunity to discuss his feelings with a calm person."

> Basic Nursing, A Psychophysiologic Approach, Sorensen and Luckmann, W.B. Saunders Company 1979, page 124

Patients with anxiety may send you messages because they are worried and they may say things that seem odd but no harm is intended. If you sense "worry" in what they said it is better to respond quickly. Send them a message right back saying, "Its okay. I'm not offended. You don't have to be scared. I'm alright and I'm not going to disown you for what you said." If you don't they will send you a slew of other messages trying to explain the one thing they thought might offend you.

If I were the patient I would think, *"What a relief! You were okay after all. I don't have to send many more messages to you to explain why I said what I said because you already understand and you're still okay with me... You understand and you still like me and you're still okay. You weren't offended after all."*

"The hallmark of a truly professional nurse is not merely her ability to take care of patients whom she personally likes and whose pleasant moods and behaviors make her feel good. The professional nurse has the ability to also care for, and about, those patients (often called "difficult") whom she may find personally upsetting."

> Basic Nursing, A Psychophysiologic Approach, Sorensen and Luckmann, W.B. Saunders Company 1979, page 133

"Illness also makes patients feel helpless, and they worry about what will happen to them in their hopeless state."

> Basic Nursing, A Psychophysiologic Approach, Sorensen and Luckmann, W.B. Saunders Company 1979, page 158

I had this really bad dream that my family doctor got a call from the hospital saying they got Medicare to approve them doing the Doppler Echocardiogram with IV insertion, Blood gas blood tests, and a Bubble test. In my dream my doctor tried to advocate for me to the hospital but they were not willing to meet all my needs. I dreamed she called me and told me they wanted to see me and she was very quick to call me because she actually called the next morning and said, "The hospital called me and said they approved that test and they really want you to do this soon. They told me, 'There were certain things they would not be able to do for you that you wanted them to do but that I need you to bite the bullet okay. I really think your doctor is on to something and I really think you need to do this so I really want you to do this okay. I really think this may be what the problem is you've been trying to tell us you thought you had all this time and I want you to find out for sure. I really need you to do this because I really think this is what it is.' In my dream, my doctor didn't even say what things they weren't going to do. Was I was going to get a man, or did they insisted I was going to get a serious trended female nurse to do the test because they weren't going to give me a chipper acting, cheery female nurse, or whether the cheery female nurses were not going to rub my head to calm me down through the IV stick and give me hugs.

In my dream I said, "No! I'm not doing it! I really want to do this test but I'm only going to do it if they meet my needs. If they don't do it, I'm not going."

In my dream, my doctor was very nice about it and we were still friends and everything was still okay, but she still acted like she wanted me to go because she thought this was the best she was going to get anybody to do for me.

I want everybody to know I am serious. Even if it is an emergency if my needs are not met I'm not going to be sticking around. I'm glad she already knows that and understands.

The people at the hospital never said they wouldn't do all this stuff for me. My wife, Bertha Marie already talked to one person and they talked like they would have no problem meeting my needs when she got through with them. The people doing the test might have not understood all of it but they were probably going to do whatever it is I wanted anyway if they thought it was what I needed so I'm glad it was just a bad dream. When people refuse to meet any of these needs it is like a nightmare to me. I have to be able to have comforting hugs, chipper acting, and cheery female nurses only to rub my head to calm me down and hold my hand through IV sticks, blood tests, and shots. I cannot have any male nurses or techs or serious trended female nurses or techs present. They all have to be chipper acting cheery female nurses only and that includes the techs and they have to be the ones to do the comforting. This is what I need and nothing else will do.

I finally got to do this test I was worried about, got the chipper acting female nurses I wanted and they gave me hugs and rubbed my head to calm me down and held my hand through the IV stick just like I asked them to and everything went very well. They put it in my chart to give me the same two girls every time I have to go to Radiology for any invasive test. I was really happy about it. My nightmare did not come true after all. Everything went very well when I went for this test. I am so thankful they were so nice to me and understood me. I really appreciate it more than they will ever know.

"Every attempt must be made to help the patient to feel and to be safe and secure."
> Basic Nursing, A Psychophysiologic Approach, Sorensen and Luckmann, W.B. Saunders Company 1979, page 158

"Patients fear being abandoned by loved ones during their illness."
>   Basic Nursing, A Psychophysiologic Approach, Sorensen
>   and Luckmann, W.B. Saunders Company 1979, page 159

"Staff members are needed to contribute to the ever-present needs
for safety, security, love, and belonging that continue into a
patient's existence in a care facility."
>   Basic Nursing, A Psychophysiologic Approach, Sorensen
>   and Luckmann, W.B. Saunders Company 1979, page 159

"In these settings staff members may be with a patient more than
loved ones are; also, they are often with him during "crisis
moments" in his life and illness when loved ones may be excluded
from his presence, e.g., surgery, intensive care, isolation and
emergencies."
>   Basic Nursing, A Psychophysiologic Approach, Sorensen
>   and Luckmann, W.B. Saunders Company 1979, page 159

The patient may call your office asking for you to advocate for
them to a nurse at a specialist's office. They want to make sure
you do everything you can possibly can. If the patient is told that
they will send their information to the specialist's office, it might
make the patient feel somewhat better. However, the anxious
patient might still fear that the specialist's office staff and nurses
might not have a complete understanding of what is going on. The
patient may fear that if you don't also talk to the staff and nurses at
that specialist's office they still might not understand the patient.
They need to have their needs explained to the people working
with them. It is also beneficial if they are given an idea as to their
personality so that they will know how best to deal with the
patient. This will reduce their anxiety considerably as well as
reassure the patient.

Instead of getting frustrated with a patient for calling your office
over and over because of the same issue, show compassion for the
patient and put yourself in their shoes. Simply give them a quick
call to reassure them that their accommodations will be met. Then
the patient can be at peace about what is about to happen.

People with anxiety problems get overwhelmed they are not able to handle the suspense of what is about to happen to them. By simply making the time to advocate for the patient this will reduce their anxiety and build much needed confidence in you as their care taker.

It is extremely important to thoroughly explain all aspects of what they will be experiencing as well as the procedure itself. The less you prolong the suspense for your patient over what is about to happen to them the better it will be for both you and them.

My needs in the medical field are always the same. It doesn't matter if I am in the doctor's office, the hospital, the dentist office, a specialist or any where.

I need chipper acting female nurses only. No male nurses or techs. Preferably a female doctor or nurse, but if the doctor is laid back it is okay if they are a male, but if they have a female APN I can go to the rest of the time I would be more comfortable with this. I need to be able to get hugs from all the staff and nurses, especially the nurses. I need a chipper acting female nurse to rub my head to calm me down and hold my hand while another chipper acting female nurse does the IV stick, Blood Test, or Shot. This has always worked really well for me. I still get panicked and sometimes even still scream, but at least it helps and makes me feel calmer than I would feel. I also need to be able to put Lidocaine/Prilocaine 2.5% cream on the site of the stick one hour before being stuck. I need completely knocked out for all invasive procedures and all the surgery room or procedure room people working with me need to be chipper acting female nurses only.

Go by this exact same list and do all of the same above things for me, especially when I am being stuck with needles or get scared over things. This list goes for the office and the procedure room people. And, the anesthesiologist cannot be a man. They have to be a woman.

Brian Evans

The chipper acting female nurse needs to do the IV stick for the procedure. If there is no female anesthesiologist, the man needs to give a chipper acting female nurse instructions on how to insert the IV and what he wants put in it to put me to sleep. Plus, I need the gas, and if at all possible, before the IV. If I can't be totally knocked out with the gas first and they put the IV in shortly after they start the gas, just make sure I am numb and woozy before you stick me. You still have to rub my head to calm me down and hold my hand when you do it and be willing to give me reassuring hugs even if they do it this way. If you don't, I won't be sticking around because I cannot handle it either way, and I cannot handle being shown impersonal care.

I'm glad I have found quotes out of your books that state that other patients are afraid of receiving impersonal care too. I like the way they state you are supposed to meet them with the personal care they need because that confirms my theory I always understood that the nurses are supposed to meet the emotional needs of the patient as well as their physical needs.

If you look in your books you will also see "touch" and "touch therapy" and "bonding with the nurse" are things that are mentioned as things of importance in your books several times over. Please meet my needs when I come your way and be my "mother surrogates" you are supposed to be for me. Thanks. Keep reading.

"A patient is not truly "taken care of" unless the nurse helps him to feel safe, secure, loved, and as one who "belongs" rather than as an outsider who is viewed as an intruder."
> Basic Nursing, A Psychophysiologic Approach, Sorensen and Luckmann, W.B. Saunders Company 1979, page 159

I need to be able to feel safe, secure and loved by you as my nurses. The cheery female nurses need to be willing to give me reassuring hugs exactly like you would a frightened child to bring me comfort. I need a cheery nurse to rub my head to calm me down and hold my hand through needle sticks of any kind.

"Patients worry about being treated impersonally. A touch of the hand, a stroke on the brow, a look, a pat, the way a patient is handled, made comfortable, and helped can all contribute to making him feel valued and close to those caring for him."

> Basic Nursing, A Psychophysiologic Approach, Sorensen and Luckmann, W.B. Saunders Company 1979, page 159

I'm always afraid of being treated impersonally. I had a hospital that did this for me for 10 years that it worked wonderful with until they got all new nurses that were standoffish. All these new nurses decided it was not in their job description to comfort their patients. Now I'm going somewhere else hoping for the same loving care I had before everything went sour at the other hospital. I was devastated when all my favorite nurses quit their jobs that understood me and they hired all these stoic acting ones to take their place that didn't understand. I need you to be like the nurses that did understand me and did meet my needs well.

"If a patient's needs for love, closeness and belonging are relatively satisfied through the concern and interest of health care personnel, then he has also been helped to meet another group of needs: the needs for esteem and self-esteem. Because he receives love, concern and respect from others, and because he feels he "belongs" and "is one" with others, the patient's feelings of self-esteem are enhanced. He is important enough that others care about "his feelings". He is not overlooked or impersonally treated as if he is merely one person out of many whose weight will leave an indistinguishable imprint on the mattress he lies on; he does not feel forgotten before he has even left the care facility. The person who has an appropriate sense of esteem feels that he is regarded by others as an individual of worth and value, and he also has these feelings about himself."

> Basic Nursing, A Psychophysiologic Approach, Sorensen and Luckmann, W.B. Saunders Company 1979, page159

I desperately need all this from you. I may appear normal to everyone because I was normalized for so many years after being taken out of special Ed.

 I am actually a special needs person, who appears to have it together, but in reality I have many dependency needs and a dire need for affection and comfort from my nurses just as I always have from birth until the present. I need you to meet those emotional needs for comfort and reassurance.

I was very disturbed by what I was told by one of my neighbors that used to be a C N A for a nursing home. This lady's boss told her, "Do not to touch your patients! Do not to get close to them! Do not call them honey! Do not to get attached to them!" She did anyway. When this C N A began to cry after bad news from the patient because they were dying or had cancer, her boss immediately got her attention and said, "That's enough! You need to go!" Because of this the C N A quit her job because she was mad. I want you to know I think this was totally uncalled for and the boss of this lady who told her this ought to be ashamed of her self. Those people are our elders and you need to be willing to take care of your elders and show them your love. Those people are your elders and they need your love and your comfort. Give it to them.

"Illness can markedly interfere with the gratifications of esteem needs. The ill person often does not feel that he is of worth and value to others, or to himself, but instead he feels he is a "drag on life," a burden, and an unpleasant reminder of those aspects of life that people prefer not to think about. All these feelings create intense worries."

> Basic Nursing, A Psychophysiologic Approach, Sorensen and Luckmann, W.B. Saunders Company 1979, page 159

"Excessive anxiety, which pain or the threat of pain often produces, must be reduced or attenuated, since it can lower a patient's pain reaction threshold and trigger systemic responses that make pain hard to combat. Generally, the more severe a person's anxiety is, the greater will be is overreaction to pain stimulation."

> Basic Nursing, A Psychophysiologic Approach, Sorensen and Luckmann, W.B. Saunders Company 1979, page 845

Brian Evans

I have a very high oversensitivity to pain. A shot and a blood test feel like being stabbed with a steak knife to me. An IV feels like being stabbed with a butcher knife to me. And, a catheter feels like a sword being run through me when you insert it in me.

"One way in which anxiety can be reduced or perhaps eliminated is by the establishment of goals that are attainable. Often patients need the assistance of a nurse to do this. First, the patients must recognize that they are anxious. This is best done in an "atmosphere of warmth and trust". Sometimes patients who are anxious react negatively toward nurses as a manifestation of their personal frustration. It is important that a nurse understand this and react to the behavior in an unanxious manner."
> Fundamentals of Nursing, Concepts and Procedures, Barbara Kozier, BSN, RN, MN and Glenora Lea Erb, BSN, RN, Addison Wesley Publishing Company, 1979, page 797

This definitely helps me.

When a nurse shows me she really cares about me and my feelings it results in an atmosphere of warmth and trust. When a nurse is nice to me by speaking gentle and calming words it always makes me feel better. I need to be reassured that everything is going to be alright in order to effectively deal with my anxiety over medical procedures. I have a dire need to receive lots of hugs from everyone dealing with me in order to stay calm.

"After patients have agreed that they are anxious, it is important to discuss all possible reasons for their anxiety. If patients can identify the cause of their anxiety, they will find it helpful to explore the case, with the objective of learning better coping mechanisms. They may see that they have overestimated the threat or that they can reduce the source of the threat by a specific action (for example, asking a teacher whether one is failing.)"
> Fundamentals of Nursing, Concepts and Procedures, Barbara Kozier, BSN, RN, MN and Glenora Lea Erb, BSN, RN, Addison Wesley Publishing Company, 1979, page 797

I switched medical insurance once trying to get a better deal. Come to find out it wasn't a great deal after all so I switched back. A few months later I got a statement stating a bill was not going to be covered by my current insurance which caused an emotional meltdown. When I called I couldn't remember all the information I needed to tell my doctor in order for her to be paid. Because I was so nervous I ended up calling her several times because I wanted her to get paid what she was supposed to be paid.

My doctor was very patient with me and even took out several minutes to help me understand that it wasn't nearly as worrisome as I had thought it to be. My reaction to her not being paid is typical with any patient that suffers with Anxiety problems. Even some normal people might get worked up over something like this.

"By personalizing nursing care, patients can feel important and that they do have control. Calling patients by name, being interested in them, and demonstrating concern about matters that patients are concerned with assist them to maintain a feeling of control over themselves and the events that affect them."

>Fundamentals of Nursing, Concepts and Procedures, Barbara Kozier, BSN, RN, MN and Glenora Lea Erb, BSN, RN, Addison Wesley Publishing Company, 1979, page 797

My doctor almost offered to allow me to take a blood test a month earlier because I was so anxious about it. If it weren't for the fact that diabetes runs in my family I would have done it but I was working hard to lose some weight because I didn't want to have to be put on medication for diabetes. Because of my fear of needles I have a major fear of having to prick myself several times a day in order to check my blood sugar levels so I backed out. My anxiety kicked into overdrive. I got all worked up over having to wait for the blood test for an entire month. It was driving me crazy. I was frantic so I begged over and over if she would just go ahead and do it. My wife, Bertha Marie, said we should wait to lose as much weight as possible before having another blood test. I was scared about not getting my needs met the second time because other doctors have made promises they didn't keep.

I needed to see for myself that my doctor would pull through for me.

After the longest month of my life my doctor did pull through. I sighed in relief when everything worked out perfectly. I gain more and more confidence with each visit because she has proven that she will always meet my needs. The only thing is they were not able to schedule a follow up appointment until five days later.

People with anxiety have an extremely hard time waiting for things to happen. If they are me they may not be able to take medicine to help deal with their anxiety. You can expect to receive several calls and/or several messages bugging you to death until the procedure takes place.

We don't mean to do this to you. It's best for everyone if you schedule the follow up appointment on that day because having to wait will cause us to worry and we will drive you crazy.

My wife had an allergy problem. She called the doctor and was told what medicine to get at the store, I automatically thought, *"Oh no! My doctor backed out of seeing you because she doesn't want to have anything to do with me anymore! When everything turns out okay, they're going to tell me they never want to see me again."*

However, if a follow up appointment had been set up I would have been relieved. I would have been assured that if something came up I could just call my doctor and they would get me in. I would feel like "What a relief! Everything's okay! They're okay with me after all. They still like me! They don't want to get rid of me! They're okay!"

You see the whole reason for the whole mess in the first place, where I drove them crazy, was I felt like I was being punished like they didn't want to see me. I felt like I was being told not to bug them anymore. The results I needed to hear did not take place quickly enough.

Brian Evans

21

The longer I had to wait to hear it, the more I thought something was wrong for sure! I needed to be assured the minute I thought something was wrong with something like, "Brian, its okay, everything's alright. I'm not upset. Everything is going to be the same as it was." I would have figured out I never offended anyone in the first place. Even if I did say something that sounded strange to my doctor, I would know that she was not going to let it get to her. We are still friends. I would not have been scared. I would have known she was still okay and would see me again.

People with anxiety need to be consoled on the spot the minute the "worry" kicks in before their imagination runs away with them. They will automatically think about all the horrible things they think you're going to think of them for something they may have said. Chances are, you may not even be upset about anything to begin with? Even if you are, it doesn't mean you are going to disown them for it.

In order to help them combat their anxiety they need to here it from you. Don't wait until they've sent 10 or 15 messages trying to explain themselves away for the message they fear you've mistaken.

"By the nurses conveying caring and understanding of their positions, the nurse can assist patients to reduce their stress. To feel that there is someone else who helps and cares is supportive to people who are stressed. Often families require time to ventilate their worries and their anxieties in order to feel assured and less stressed. The patient is provided with time to ventilate his or her feelings and thoughts. As part of the plan of care, nurses need to allow for time for patients to describe their feelings and worries if they wish. Some people find it relatively easy to describe their feelings, while others may prove hesitant to do so. The nurses need to be sensitive to the patient's needs and neither to probe with questions nor be too busy to listen."

Fundamentals of Nursing, Concepts and Procedures, Barbara Kozier, BSN, RN, MN and Glenora Lea Erb, BSN, RN, Addison Wesley Publishing Company, 1979, page 132

"Older adults with depression and anxiety are less likely than young adults to be accurately diagnosed (Varcarolis and others, 2006)."

> Fundamentals of Nursing, 7th Edition, Potter and Perry, Mosby Elsevier, 2009, page 491

"Anxiety – mental uneasiness owing to an impending or anticipated threat often associated with physiologic changes such as increase pulse rate or sweating"

> Fundamentals of Nursing, Concepts and Procedures, Barbara Kozier and Glenora Lea Erb, Addison-Wesley Publishing Company, 1979, page 929

Here are the best ways to handle me with my anxiety issues:

1. Make follow up appointments as close together as possible
2. Make sure to respond as quickly as possible to any phone messages, face book messages or emails I may send you
3. Assure me you got the message when I call you
4. Answer any medical questions I need answered as promptly as possible
5. Let me know you are not offended about something anything I may have said or written
6. Let me know everything is still okay and we are still friends

> There are going to be times when this happens with any disabled person. They were probably just being a kid at heart when they said or asked you whatever odd thing they said and meant nothing mischievous whatsoever. What they wanted from you that they asked of you came from the heart of a little child rather than a normal adult. Please remember this when dealing with Autistic people and other disabled people with disabilities similar to that of mental retardation. Even though I have high functioning autism I still have areas of mental retardation but just not enough to give me a mentally retarded score in those areas.

When I say, do or ask odd things please remember, a normal adult didn't say, do or ask the odd things. A child inside an adult body made this request to you or said this to you out of a childlike heart with totally innocent motives. Please keep this in mind when dealing with the disabled community. Thanks.

7. Try not to prolong suspense about anything that has to do with appointments, medical questions or advocacy. I need to know the details of who, what, when, where, why, how, will you advocate for me?

I get extremely anxious wondering if people who read my book will be offended or be compassionately understanding. I feel like I have to explain myself thoroughly because I don't want to offend anyone. I just want to help them understand me.

When I am in the hospital I am terrified so I need my nurses and people dealing with me to be kind and give me personalized care. In order to keep me calm I need the nurses to frequently give me comforting hugs like they would a terrified child. I only want chipper acting female nurses because men and grumpy female nurses tortured me as a child in medical settings.

I also need for them to rub my head to calm me down and hold my hand through any needle sticks, blood tests, IVs, shots, blades, and scalpels, anything sharp or scary, even tube insertions as well as removal of these items. Please only do tube insertions when I am completely knocked out, even if it is a urinary catheter or laryngoscope, or the like.

When I am in the hospital and my nurse is called to another floor it is very important that they tell me when they leave. If I am left in the dark and I wonder where they went I will have an emotional meltdown. If they show up a couple hours later I will have been under stress and worried the entire time which would not be good for my healing process.

I just need to receive a lot of tender loving care and affection. I need to be pampered by chipper acting female nurses with motherly personalities who will treat me like I am their own little boy. I know this may sound strange to you, but because of my autism, this is what I need. Thank you.

"Anxiety disorders are the most prevalent disorders in later life and are continuations of life-long illnesses (Hyer and Sohnle, 2001)"
> Fundamentals of Nursing, 7th Edition, Potter and Perry, Mosby Elsevier, 2009, page 491

"Often the client has difficulty expressing exactly what is most bothersome about the situation until there is an opportunity to discuss it with someone who has time to listen."
> Fundamentals of Nursing, 7th Edition, Potter and Perry, Mosby Elsevier, 2009, page 492

This has always been a very big problem for me. When nurses don't want to listen, or I can't get what I'm wanting to say from my head out my mouth I may bug them several times trying desperately to get them to understand. When I finally do get through, they turn the cold shoulder on me and act like, "Don't bug me anymore. I'm tired of hearing about it. I don't want to talk to you about it anymore."

Apparently this must happen with other patients to for a comment like this one to be in their nursing books.

"When stress overwhelms a person's existing coping mechanisms, disequilibrium occurs, and a crisis results (Aguilera, 1998). If symptoms of stress persist beyond the duration of the sensor, a person has experienced trauma (Hyer and Sohnle, 2001)"
> Fundamentals of Nursing, 7th Edition, Potter and Perry, Mosby Elsevier, 2009, page 486

It is very important to keep in mind why you chose to be a nurse; to help comfort the people in your care and not for the check.

Nurses do not make near enough money for that to be the reason for sure. Also keep in mind that each person is different and may be comforted by different things. Never assume that the way that you want to bring comfort is what will work, I have special needs that are not exactly like anyone else. When my need for comfort is not met I am overwhelmed with feelings of hopelessness.

I am careful to be sure everyone who deals with me has my list of needs before anything is done. These are genuine needs that need to be met I cannot handle it any other way. That includes my need for the hugs, the head rubs and the hand holds, and the need for chipper acting, cheery female nurses and techs only.

If you can arrange for these needs to be met, then that's great. If not, I know I have the right to refuse care so I will not be sticking around for you to do anything to me. That's just the way it is.

"Crisis differs from stress in the degree of severity, although there are many similarities between stress and crisis. A client who perceives a situation as stressful, who is unable to cope in any ways that have worked before, and who has insufficient supports is experiencing a crisis. A crisis is devastating and requires use of all recourses available (Aguilera, 1998.) Unlike stress, which ends when the stressor is gone, the effects of a trauma last for years (Hyer and Sohnle, 2001)."

> Fundamentals of Nursing, 7th Edition, Potter and Perry, Mosby Elsevier, 2009, page 493

I have had many bad experiences in the medical field throughout my lifetime which has resulted in major trauma. The trauma from how I have been treated by past still affects me. I am usually fearful of how I will be treated, even if they are someone I love and trust. Because of broken promises to meet my needs at other doctor's offices, whether I really believed it to be true in my heart or not, I thought that the same thing could happen with the doctor I go to now. In my heart I felt like I knew this was not true. But because I have been burned so many times before I still genuinely feared the past would repeat itself.

My heart felt belief was my own sweet caring doctor would never do such a thing. I wasn't completely convinced until, she met all my needs for blood test twice. As a result, I feel like I have driven her up the wall over this until I got to see for myself that in fact she would pull through for me a second time. I am very happy with her and am sorry for letting my fears of being disappointed cause me to be a nuisance.

She is the most wonderful doctor I have ever had and the sweetest doctor I've ever known and I greatly appreciate everything she has ever done for me.

"A nurse's moods and behaviors may actually increase the suffering of some patients physically as well as psychologically and may delay their recovery." What behavioral qualities might patients find helpful in a nurse? Frequently people who are ill want to be cared for by a person, who is accepting, thoughtful, gentle, nurturing, kind, genuine, emotionally warm, caring, and giving. Often it helps the person to relax and feel better if his needs can be anticipated by others. Nursing requires the abilities to listen carefully to patients and to accept them during both pleasant and unpleasant moments. The nurse who listens attentively allows the patient to put his feelings into words. The nurse also coveys to the patient the feeling that she will consider and respond to anything the patient has to say and that she will try to talk with the patient about anything he wishes to discuss. In other words, the helpful nurse's words and behaviors convey to the patient that his verbal and nonverbal expressions of his thoughts and feelings will not be devastating to her or provoke in her behaviors that are not in the patient's best interests. The nurse demonstrates to the patient that she is able to (a) hear what they patient has to say, (b) consider and respond to the patient's words, and (c) notice and consider the patient's appearance and actions (physical condition and nonverbal behaviors) and respond in helpful ways."

> Basic Nursing: A Psychophysiologic Approach, Sorensen and Luckmann, W. B. Saunders Company, 1979, page 132

"At times, a nurse may feel a sense of discomfort in response to what a patient is saying or the specific manner in which he is acting, however, she still strives to convey a general acceptance of the patient as a person. That is to say, the attitude the nurse tries to convey to the patient is: "I care about you even though these particular words or this specific behavior of yours makes me uncomfortable."

> Basic Nursing: A Psychophysiologic Approach, Sorensen and Luckmann, W. B. Saunders Company, 1979, page 132

"This acceptance of the patient as a person requires that the nurse demonstrated a genuine appreciation of the patient's situation rather than only looking at his behavior by itself and reacting to it without attempting to understand what prompts the behavior."

> Basic Nursing: A Psychophysiologic Approach, Sorensen and Luckmann, W. B. Saunders Company, 1979, page 132

"Many times an anxious patient needs repeated explanations of what is happening to him, as well as repeated reassurances that you are trying to help him."

> Giving Emergency Care Competently, page 41, Nursing Skillbook, Intermed Communications, Inc., 1979

"Help others cope with stress by showing how much you appreciate them."

> Giving Emergency Care Competently, page 23, Nursing Skillbook, Intermed Communications, Inc., 1979

"A good triage nurse provides emotional support to the patient's family."

> Giving Emergency Care Competently, page 23, Nursing Skillbook, Intermed Communications, Inc., 1979

"A lady nurse standing next to a female patient in distress puts her arm around her and looks at her with concern in the picture of this book."

> Giving Emergency Care Competently, page 23, Nursing Skillbook, Intermed Communications Inc., 1979

"In maintaining good public relations, inform members of the patient's family about his condition and comfort him."
>   Giving Emergency Care Competently, page 20, Nursing
>   Skillbook, Intermed Communications, Inc., 1979

"Whenever you talk to a patient treat him as you would like to be treated if you were in the same circumstances."
>   Giving Emergency Care Competently, page 20, Nursing
>   Skillbook, Intermed Communications, Inc., 1979

"So do what you can to alleviate his anxiety. Speak to him slowly and calmly. Encourage him to express his feelings to you and then listen."
>   Giving Emergency Care Competently, page 41, Nursing
>   Skillbook, 1979

"Give the patient emotional support and reassurance."
>   Giving Emergency Care Competently, page 41, Nursing
>   Skillbook, Intermed Communications, Inc., 1979

"When something interferes with a person's ability to maintain his equilibrium, he feels threatened. In some cases, he may even feel threatened by something he anticipates for example, impending surgery."
>   Using Crisis Intervention Wisely, page 16, Nursing Skillbook,
>   Intermed Communications, Inc., 1975

"Watch for the patient faced with a stressful situation. He may take the steps which lead to crisis."
>   Using Crisis Intervention Wisely, page 16, Nursing
>   Skillbook, Intermed Communications, Inc., 1975

"Try to understand why your patient's behaving the way he is, and strive to accept him. Any negative feelings you show toward him will add to his stress. What's more you can't assess a patient's stress level accurately if your own feelings interfere. You're sure to react differently, even though you may not realize it."

 Using Crisis Intervention Wisely, pages 18&19, Nursing Skillbook, Intermed Communications, Inc., 1975

My needs may be odd to some people but the need for comfort and care should be met freely.

"A patient who says he has a problem deserves your attention, no matter how insignificant that problem may seem to you."

 Using Crisis Intervention Wisely, pages 20&21, Nursing Skillbook, Intermed Communications, Inc., 1975

I have had doctors I really wanted to see badly that blew me off because they really didn't think my problem was bad enough to see me about. When they do it makes me worry that there might be something wrong where they really don't want to see me unless they just absolutely have to because they feel I've annoyed them or offended them in some way or another.

"When someone is in severe stress, even a trivial incident can throw him into crisis."

 Using Crisis Intervention Wisely, page 21, Nursing Skillbook, Intermed Communications, Inc., 1975

When I am really worked up about something already and I worry that someone has a misunderstood something I said or did, I get even more anxious. I usually get myself worked up into a panic.

"To differentiate between a patient who's effectively coping with severe stress, one who's heading for a crisis, and one who's already in crisis, complete the following steps: (1) investigate unusual behavior, (2) look for a trigger event, and (3) determine how involved the patient is with his problem."

> Using Crisis Intervention Wisely, page 18, Nursing Skills Book, 1975

"Being hospitalized or bringing a loved one to the hospital is a stressful event for most people. However, no one can predict how each person will perceive the event, or if he can cope with it successfully. He may do reasonably well at first, then falter under added stress. Or he may start out poorly, then develop new coping mechanisms that help him adapt to his situation. You'll get your first impression of your patient's coping abilities when you do your initial assessment. At that time, watch for physical and psychologic clues that he's under severe stress. Investigate anything unusual. Try to find out what's normal for your patient. Try to understand why he is behaving the way he is and strive to accept him."

> Using Crisis Intervention Wisely, page 18, Nursing Skills Book, Intermed Communications, Inc., 1975

"By listening to the patient in tears or providing support or solitude, you can help ease his stress and perhaps avert a crisis."

> Using Crisis Intervention Wisely, page 18, Nursing Skills Book, Intermed Communications, Inc., 1975

"Let's go immediately to the next step: identifying and relieving the patient's most pressing problem. To illustrate, think back to the claustrophobic patient in that chapter. From the time of admission his stress level escalated rapidly. Then he went into a full-blown crisis when the nurse raised his side rails. What's his most pressing problem at that point? His difficulties adjusting to hospitalization? No, it's the raised side rails, because that's what triggered his panic. Before you can help him adjust to hospitalization, you must do something about his immediate problem. Lower both side rails, or at least one of them.

Stay with him after that so you can establish a rapport that'll help you discover what's behind the crisis. And, you can plan further interventions to relieve much of the stress he feels from hospitalization. When you sense an impending crisis- or know that one exists – don't waist precious time trying to thoroughly analyze the situation. Calm the patient as quickly as possible."

> Using Crisis Intervention Wisely, pages 26&28,
> Nursing Skills Book, Intermed Communications, Inc., 1975

"Autism in all its forms is a complex, lifelong neurodevelopmental disorder that can profoundly affect a person's ability to communicate with, and understand the behaviors of those around them. People with autism find it difficult to communicate their thoughts, feelings, and physical sensations in ways that are easy for others to understand; this can render them very vulnerable when illness strikes, or when normal physical development demands attention."

> Health Care and the Autism Spectrum, A Guide to Health
> Professionals, Parents, and Carers, Alison Morton-Cooper,
> Jessica Kingsley Publishers, 2004, page 22

"For the person affected by autism, even a typical family doctor consultation or visit to the practice nurse can be a traumatic and anxiety-provoking experience with unintended outcomes for those involved."

> Health Care and the Autism Spectrum, A Guide to Health
> Professionals, Parents, and Carers, Alison Morton-Cooper,
> Jessica Kingsley Publishers, 2004, page 23

I really like my family doctor a great deal and I worry myself sick that I might say or do something that may offend her. If I don't get sick and have to wait a very long time before my next appointment the added suspense increases my anxiety over a period of time until it builds into a panic situation. It is very traumatic for me. I know I need to be reassured immediately that everything is okay or I will drive my wife and her absolutely crazy until my doctor reassures me.

When I sense aggravation over how much I messaged or called my doctor before I finally get a word of reassurance, the reassurance is harder to grasp. Had I been reassured sooner, as soon as my doctor picked up on my worry I would feel immediately relieved on the spot. It doesn't occur to me that if I call on Friday it is impossible to hear from her till Monday. I am trying to call when I know they are open to save myself from leaving so many messages.

"The risks involved are very real. First there is the risk that the patient may be misunderstood or have their needs misinterpreted. Then there is the risk of misdiagnosis resulting from poor-quality communication."
> Health Care and the Autism Spectrum, A Guide to Health Professionals, Parents, and Carers, Alison Morton-Cooper, Jessica Kingsley Publishers, 2004, page 23

My needs are constantly misinterpreted by other doctors and nurses. My newest family doctor however, is very understanding of my special needs for comfort and care in nursing. Not only does she meet them herself but advocates for me to others so they will do the same thing.

"The pressures and stresses of 'trying to be normal' re-emerge, placing the child, young person or adult under yet more strain, with the risk of regression into withdrawal and the development of depression and anxiety disorders."
> Health Care and the Autism Spectrum, A Guide to Health Professionals, Parents, and Carers, Alison Morton-Cooper, Jessica Kingsley Publishers, 2004, page 27

I have felt a great deal of pressure my entire life to meet up to the expectations of the normal world after being taken out of Special Ed. People expect more of me than what I can give because they think I am normal. I only appear normal to them because I was normalized by the school system. But I still have the same childlike emotional needs I had when I was in Special Ed and they still need met by those taking care of me, especially nurses.

"Professionals and the public need to understand that autism is lifelong even where it outwardly appears to be 'mild'. Support services and understanding need to be built around this."

> Health Care and the Autism Spectrum, A Guide to Health Professionals, Parents, and Carers, Alison Morton-Cooper, Jessica Kingsley Publishers, 2004, page 27

Some people think people grow out of Autism but that is simply not true. I have always been autistic and have had the same special needs and sensory issues I always had since birth. The only difference is I grew out of some of the erratic symptoms like screaming constantly. The autism is always there and always will be for life.

"Emotional support for all people with autism begins with trying to gain an understanding of what the world is like from their perspective."

> Health Care and the Autism Spectrum, A Guide to Health Professionals, Parents, and Carers, Alison Morton-Cooper, Jessica Kingsley Publishers, 2004, page 27

I have a different perspective than people of the normal world. I see things like a child would see them. I have the needs of a child. Some of my interests are things that would not interest the average man, for instance I like Victorian dolls. I even got a Princessopoly board game, a "Princess and the Pauper" movie and other kid movies, and a Candy Land board game for Christmas as well as more dolls, more candles, more flavor scented body wash, more flavor scented bath salts, more flavor scented soap, more Christmas records, three Sandra Kuck kid calendars, a flower calendar, and a few others, plus the ones I made myself of landscapes of flowers, and, I got coloring books. I got a slew of these kinds of gifts. Does this sound like the typical guy to you? I want you to see who I really am and what I am really like. I want you to see the real me.

One of my guy friends was giving me a hard time about my manhood and I was thinking, "I really don't care anything about my manhood. I don't care about things like that. That's just not me." He really didn't know a whole lot about me. He'd only seen me a few times so he hadn't figured it out yet. I think he figured that out now.

You're probably thinking, "I thought you said you didn't like guys and only hang around girls."

That's true. I do have a few guy friends but I really don't hang around them very much because I like to be with girls better. I relate better to other ladies and girls and I have more of their interests than I do guys, and I'm a lot like a kid. Most of the people I hang around most of the time are ladies. I really don't care for men that much. I'm more of a girly guy that acts more like a kid than a man.

I even read a Couple's devotional book that had biography stories below the verses. I normally like those, but I kept reading stuff about men. I really don't care for those. It was men this, men that, and men think this and men like that, and I actually got upset and felt depressed fearing that's the way people thought I was just because this is what was typical and I thought, "Will you leave me alone?! I'm not like you!"

When I read this I thought, "First this guy, now this book. Does everybody have to shove men in my face and assume I act like men when I don't even think anything like men think?"

It wasn't the verses that upset me. I always like the verses. I just didn't like the stories about the men because it was just another reminder that I'm different and people don't think like me. In one story they said something about men that typically gave their spouses massages as a precursor to sex.

I was upset and I thought, "That's not the reason I give my wife a foot massage! That's not the reason I ever liked to give a lady a foot massage! I like ladies' feet and I like to rub them or pet them, but all it does for me is make me feel like I pet a cat. It feels soft on my hands and it relaxes me! That's all! To me a foot massage is a foot massage! And, to me a massage is a massage and is separate from any type of sexual advances!"

After I saw this, I thought, "I suppose everyone else thinks I think this way just because these men think this way! I'm not like other men! I'm tired of being judged for what other men think when I don't think like they do! There are things I want for reasons that are not the same as other men! When I give a massage I don't do it for the same reason as them! I'm not that way! I don't think like them!" There are things that I wish I could do or ask for that I always have to worry about asking for all because "men" have a different reason for doing everything than I do with practically everything. We don't think the same way. We don't like the same things. And, we don't have the same reasons for wanting the same things. I ask for the things I ask for out of "neediness" and they ask for it out of mischievousness. I get the feeling they meant full massages though, and that does not make me feel sexual either.

In another story they said that men typically "do not" like to do the dishes for their wives. I was mad and thought, "I love to do the dishes for my wife! What's wrong with these people anyway?! Are they too manly to wash the dishes in the house for the wife?! I always like to wash the dishes and vacuum the floor and do the laundry but, when it comes to mowing the lawn or doing a vegetable garden or fixing a sink or a car, that's a different story!" They also talked about men liking to go hunting and fishing in another story and that did not fit my personality at all. I hate hunting and fishing. I'd rather have a tea party with the ladies than go hunting or fishing with another guy. There was just one thing right after the other and everything they ever said about, "Men like this, men think like that, and men like to do the following activities" all of it was the opposite of what I am like.

Other people don't understand I don't think like typical guys so it makes me upset because they want to base judgment on everything I say or do on what the typical guy says or does when I don't think like typical guys think. I'm a child at heart. I'm a sentimentalist. Their thinking doesn't fit my thinking. I'm not like them. It wouldn't have mattered if it had been a secular book I would have felt the same way. I would have rathered just read my regular bible than to read stories about how modern day men think and act. It just makes me upset when I read other stories about men. Watching movies about how modern day men think and act toward each other also depress me. I've even seen men on some of these shows where a little boy that everyone else would have considered to be a geek was interested in their little daughter and these men would want to sternly lecture the poor little sentimentalist boy in the movie when they were interested in their daughter and wanted to let them know they'd better not make any advances toward their girl or give them cooties. When I saw these movies I thought, "Will you cut it out?! Don't you see it?! That boy is a sentimentalist. They don't think like other boys! You don't have to worry about them doing anything to your girl! Be glad they weren't a hippy with tattoos or a drunkard or a druggy, or a bully, or some rebel that goes around thinking their slicker than I'll get out! These are the ones you have to worry about! Not them! Even the wife of one of the guys on "Duck Dynasty" that a friend of ours watches said this when her husband acted like this. I also get depressed when I see the way these men react to each other in these movies because I feel totally out of place. It's so ridiculous.

And some of these modern day shows where they have a bunch of crackpot jokers for guys that egg each other on about the most ridiculous things you ever heard and think its funny make me really uncomfortable.

Now, you come up with one about the way they acted and thought in the 1800s and that's not so bad, but I still like ladies better. I'd much rather see a movie about girls and ladies better.

Brian Evans
37

I relate better to girls and ladies and kids and I want all my female nurses I want to see me as a kid. I'm tired of being punished for thinking like a man when I say childish things just because some man out there has some mischievous reason for saying and asking for the same things I do when I think like a kid. It's not my fault they have mischievous reasons for the same things I have innocent reasons for. I'm not like them. I'm an ex-Special Ed student. I'm a child in a man's body and I don't think like them at all and I will not be punished for every little thing I say or ask just because some stupid man out there wanted the same things for the wrong reasons that I wanted for the right reasons.

Stop punishing me for the way they think. I'm not them, I'm me.

Remember, just because I'm worried you will think something bad about me for something doesn't mean you have anything to worry about.

You're probably thinking, "If we don't have anything to worry about then why did it occur to you to defend yourself about such things?"

You want to know why? Because people have come up with things like this about me before suggesting I thought things I never thought just because of what the opera people in Abilene, Texas made me look like.

If people had not said things to me like the things I'm suggesting you might say to me if you got the wrong idea about me for something it wouldn't occur to me to defend myself about such things, but because they did say these things about me based on what a bunch of opera trainers made me look like it does occur to me to be worried you will think these things about me so I am still innocent.

It's not because I do think these type of thoughts that I am defending myself about how I think, but because of how I fear you will think I think about things based on how I have been judged in the past where I was constantly falsely accused of things based on some ridiculous body language I was taught to have that I was stuck looking like that these opera people caused me to look like at all times whether I liked it or not. So, as a result I was judged and everybody thought I was a womanizer and a wife beater when I was not ever since because of some stupid play I was in. I didn't even have a wife and I was not a womanizer. I just looked weird because of what these people made me look like. No one ever accused me of this kind of thing before I met these people and since I moved to Arkansas no one has here either. I never did anything to anyone and no one ever thought I did either before I met these people.

As soon as I finally managed to break free of what these opera people made me look like, that's when the kind of girls I liked began to like me again and saw me for who I really was, the real Brian Evans.

And, by the way, I finally got married years later and my wife can assure you I am no such kind of person at all.

The whole thing was completely ridiculous and I suffered traumatic damage for a decade and a half for looking like something I was not whether I was what I looked like I was or not.

If you think I'm joking, it's happened to others. There was someone on the news a year or two ago that was continually criticized by his peers because he played a bad guy in a movie and in real life he was nothing like the character he played. He was really a nice guy.

It wasn't until well after I moved to Arkansas I found out I had Autism.

My mother tried to tell my doctor at age 10 she thought I had it when she thought my behaviors matched that of kids she saw with autism on a television program about autism but he said I was too old. He said, "Oh no! He doesn't have autism. He's too old to have autism. Autism is a little kid's disease. You have a big kid." I was diagnosed with Autism at the age of 35 years and 10 months old.

Even when I used to live at home in Abilene still looking for a girlfriend at the time and having trouble finding one, my mother said, "That's just it. Girls want a man that can handle things. They want someone different from them not someone that thinks like them. That's what the problem is. You think just like them. You never did know how to handle things but you used to try, but now, you don't even try. You just let people run all over you. They don't want someone like them. You think more like girls do than you do other guys. You think too much like them and not like other guys."

When I say something odd or ask something odd I want my nurses to know I'm just being a kid and be willing to just blow it off immediately and say, "Oh, he's just being a kid." I'm not like you.

Socially and emotionally I'm a 5 year old in a man's body according to two IQ tests I had done recently.

Intellectually I'm far smarter, but socially and emotionally I'm not.

Bertha would take it a step further and say I am a 2 year old in a man's body.

I just want you to see the truth and see the light, so you don't misjudge me for silly things and will recognize all my childlike needs and realize they are real, genuine dire needs I have.

"It's amazing how quickly it is possible to establish a rapport with your patient who has an autism spectrum condition once they have come to recognize your appreciation of their difficulties and anxieties. A sound therapeutic relationship can follow that will impact on the whole family's ability to thrive and flourish, despite the sometimes gloomy predictions about how people are likely to manage aspects of their lives."

> Health Care and the Autism Spectrum, A Guide to Health Professionals, Parents, and Carers, Alison Morton-Cooper, Jessica Kingsley Publishers, 2004, page 46

"Autism is beginning to explain a good deal of the emotional and behavioral difficulties of people who in the past have been written off as extremely eccentric or rude."

> Health Care and the Autism Spectrum, A Guide to Health Professionals, Parents, and Carers, Alison Morton-Cooper, Jessica Kingsley Publishers, 2004, page 46

Many people thought I was eccentric when I was in my 20s. There may be some that still do, especially in the medical community. What they need to understand is everything about me that seems odd to them is probably coming from my autism. They also need to realize that I am like a child with childlike needs and interests.

When I say childlike things they often get misunderstood. I get judged on the basis of what an adult thinks about whatever I think, when technically, my reason for wanting the things I wish to have are for the same reason as a child. It sounds strange, but once you figure that out, you think, "He's just being a kid. Leave him be. Don't worry about it. He's just acting like a 5-year-old as usual."

"Staff working in the reception areas of hospitals should be alerted to the behaviors and needs of people with autism to a point where they can at least identify characteristic behaviors. This would reduce the potential for misunderstandings and altercations, as well as saving time and unnecessary distress for everyone involved."

> Health Care and the Autism Spectrum, A Guide to Health Professionals, Parents, and Carers, Alison Morton-Cooper, Jessica Kingsley Publishers, 2004, page 49

"Remember, too, that a proportion of people with autism will have normal or above-average intelligence (as defined by standard IQ testing). You will therefore have to exercise judgment as to the language you use do discuss any concerns or questions they may have."

> Health Care and the Autism Spectrum, A Guide to Health Professionals, Parents, and Carers, Alison Morton-Cooper, Jessica Kingsley Publishers, 2004, page 52

This is where a lot of people mess up with me. My problem is almost upside down of what I think these guys are saying here.

I have a near normal or near average intelligence in most areas but a low borderline IQ in perceptual reasoning which includes socialization, communication, performing tasks, and spatial perception problems.

Because of the higher number, people assume I can think like the normal person in every way including socially.

In fact, I tend to think like a child in the areas of socialization and communication. I'm treated harshly by others who take something I say or do of an innocent nature and turn it into a mischievous act.

They base my behavior on how the normal everyday person wants the same things for all the wrong reasons. So, as a result, when I ask for my needs to be met they think I have alterior motives. I feel like I am being scolded, punished or interrogated.

It's almost like they think if you treat average to above average autistics like normal intelligent individuals they will act like they are.

Where I am concerned, I am very intelligent in some and I want credit in these areas. Give them credit where credit is due. But in the areas of socialization and communication where I have childlike needs then they need to be met in childlike ways. I have legitimate needs for the hugs, head rubs, affection, etc. and these needs are innocent in nature. I'm like a child in a man's body and I wish to be treated that way.

I want you to see what people saw in me before being trained in the opera after I found out I had the voice in 1986.

What did I act like? I acted like a whimsical little boy. How did I pick up all these sophisticated mannerisms that make no sense to people? I was trained over and over.

Why was I got stuck acting like them? Because I have to be one way or the other, I can't act differently in different situations like most people can. I have finally managed to get most of that out of the way. Now people see the real Brian Evans. You see the personality of me before the music and opera people messed everything up for me.

I wish to be treated like my Special Ed teachers treated me back then with lots of hugs, love, compassion, affection.

When I am in a medical situation I need to have my head rubbed to calm me down and my hand held through needle sticks by chipper acting, cheery female nurses and techs only. They need to have motherly personalities, who will pamper me to death as if I was their own little boy. They also need to give me hugs and let me hug them.

You do this and we have it made.

Brian Evans
43

Believe it or not I was I.Q. tested by two different psychologists in the past year. Both of them said I had the Socialization of a 5 year old and the Communication of an 8 to 10 year old.

Most of my general intelligence was below average to near average and the rest of my scores were borderline normal. I was right above a retarded person.

When I went to college, there were actually guys that would take me to the side and say, "I hate to say this, I think your really smart and everything but I think you're sociably retarded."

My boss at Dollar General even came to me one day at my last job in Abilene, Texas and said, "Do you mind if I tell you something? You're book smart, but you're not street smart. I'm afraid someone is going to take advantage of you one of these days. I really am."

When my wife Bertha Marie was researching Autism 12 years ago we both saw something in one of the papers we printed off of the internet. Most of them were from Autistics.org, where I think this comment probably came from, but there were 3 or 4 other sites so it could have been theirs.

The comment went like this: "Autistic people may see either too immature or too mature or both. This is a common tendency with people who have autism."

When I saw that I thought, "*I would probably pass for someone that is both, because I'm immature compared to everyone else in that I think so much like a child. When it comes to things like other peers wanting to get into some kind of mischief and trying to talk me into joining them, I try to get out of it because I don't want to have any part of it. In that way, I was always more mature than most of my peers.*"

"As autism is generally accepted as a medical diagnosis, it would seem to be in the person's best interests to have whatever additional health problem they are experiencing assessed in the context of their existing disability, so that most referring physicians or health practitioners would include this information in the referring letter or documentation."

> Health Care and the Autism Spectrum, A Guide to Health Professionals, Parents, and Carers, Alison Morton-Cooper, Jessica Kingsley Publishers, 2004, page 53

"Remember that verbal responses from the person with autism may be delayed or unobtainable. You may have to interpret behavioral responses instead."

> Health Care and the Autism Spectrum, A Guide to Health Professionals, Parents, and Carers, Alison Morton-Cooper, Jessica Kingsley Publishers, 2004, page 58

"Give them time to respond and orientate themselves. Bear in mind that some may present with problems allied to their neurological vulnerability."

> Health Care and the Autism Spectrum, A Guide to Health Professionals, Parents, and Carers, Alison Morton-Cooper, Jessica Kingsley Publishers, 2004, page 58

"Be aware that one of the key problems experienced by people with autism is a failure to understand and decode facial expressions, gestures, and body language. Your usual reassuring smile may not be enough to calm them if they are feeling bewildered and unsure of what you expect from them."

> Health Care and the Autism Spectrum, A Guide to Health Professionals, Parents, and Carers, Alison Morton-Cooper, Jessica Kingsley Publishers, 2004, page 59

Sometimes I'm so nervous about what people think of me and how they will respond to me and what is about to happen to me that I don't know what to think and get all worked up about it.

"Individualize care as much as possible and, if your patient is to be admitted to the hospital, make sure at handover that as much information about the person's difficulties or sensitivities as possible is shared with ward or departmental staff (including anyone involved in diagnostic procedures, such as radiographers, or in transportation, such as porters or ambulance drivers)."

> Health Care and the Autism Spectrum, A Guide to Health Professionals, Parents, and Carers, Alison Morton-Cooper, Jessica Kingsley Publishers, 2004, page 60

"Sometimes the person will have a fear or phobia of objects or situations that prevent him or her from doing what is necessary. Bear this in mind when undertaking physical procedures or trying to obtain blood or urine samples."

> Health Care and the Autism Spectrum, A Guide to Health Professionals, Parents, and Carers, Alison Morton-Cooper, Jessica Kingsley Publishers, 2004, page 62

"Again, be aware that any variation in normal routine or surroundings may well cause your patient extreme anxiety especially if an overnight stay is involved. Find out whether anything can be done to mitigate this, either by using the patient's special interests to fill in any waiting time or by bringing in familiar or favored items from home. The more able patient with autism may appear very tense and watchful and talk at length about any worries. That's why having someone confident and experienced to stay with the patient for reassurance is so important."

> Health Care and the Autism Spectrum, A Guide to Health Professionals, Parents, and Carers, Alison Morton-Cooper, Jessica Kingsley Publishers, 2004, page 69

"Whatever the situation, staff will have to make sure that everyone involved in the patient's care is informed of the patient's particular difficulties in communicating and relating to others, and that care plans are appropriately documented with any special area of concern. It can be helpful for the hospital if relatives, or indeed the patient, bring or carry with them a leaflet giving information on the autism spectrum and how it affects people."

> Health Care and the Autism Spectrum, A Guide to Health Professionals, Parents, and Carers, Alison Morton-Cooper, Jessica Kingsley Publishers, 2004, page 72

"Nursing the patient with autism well, therefore, draws on this kind of engagement with practice and with the moral endeavor to do what is best in the interests of the patient given their needs and personal aspirations."

> Health Care and the Autism Spectrum, A Guide to Health Professionals, Parents, and Carers, Alison Morton-Cooper, Jessica Kingsley Publishers, 2004, page 85

"If catherization is required because of urinary problems or surgery, special care will be needed to see that this is carried out as gently as possible or it is likely to cause extreme distress. Similarly, any invasive procedure, such as inserting chest or wound drains or cleaning wounds and attending to pressure area care, will require very sensitive and minimal handling and close observation."

> Health Care and the Autism Spectrum, A Guide to Health Professionals, Parents, and Carers, Alison Morton-Cooper, Jessica Kingsley Publishers, 2004, page 94

"Patients will normally need to be cared for by at least two nursing staff together if they are febrile and unwell, for they may be very restless and agitated and unable to understand what is being done to help them."

> Health Care and the Autism Spectrum, A Guide to Health Professionals, Parents, and Carers, Alison Morton-Cooper, Jessica Kingsley Publishers, 2004, page 94

This is a very good idea because the greater the number of friendlier chipper acting, cheery female nurses the better. You need at least two to get me through needle sticks, IVs, Blood Tests, Shots, Biopsies, Tube Insertions, etc. If there is a tube insertion I must be put to sleep for that because I cannot handle that awake. The same goes for urinary catheters or heart catheters either one. It would prefer to be put to sleep for the IV's also, but most people won't do that, so one chipper acting female nurse needs to do the IV stick as gently as they can while another chipper acting female nurse rubs my head to calm me down and holds my hand to comfort me.

I have a severe oversensitivity to pain and a severe fear of needles and need all the help I can get.

"Carers and families need support not only during a period of hospitalization for their relative with autism, but also in day-to-day living. Staff working in community or residential settings recognize that working with people with autism can be draining, physically and emotionally, but also very rewarding. They also know, however, that (residential care workers excepted) they can go home at the end of their shift or working hours and recoup energy given up at work."

> Health Care and the Autism Spectrum, A Guide to Health
> Professionals, Parents, and Carers, Alison Morton-Cooper,
> Jessica Kingsley Publishers, 2004, page 101

"Responses to serious illness and death can depend a great deal on an individual's faith and cultural practices. "Care" and "sensitivity" will be needed by those disclosing bad news to see that the individual is properly supported and understands what is expected of them."

> Health Care and the Autism Spectrum, A Guide to Health
> Professionals, Parents, and Carers, Alison Morton-Cooper,
> Jessica Kingsley Publishers, 2004, page 105

I am very sensitive to this kind of a thing and I need your care and sensitivity and love and hugs and affection as much as possible.

Brian Evans
48

Right now I need this even more to a dramatically increased degree from what it already was because my mother is not doing too well. I am a very clingy person already. Now I am even clingier. Please be ready for this when you see me. My mother may experience death at any time. She is getting old and is only 5 years away from how old my granny was when she died. It could be anytime in the next 5 years plus or minus a year or two. But when it happens, be ready for it. I need your help something fierce because this kind of a thing is incredibly hard for me to handle. I don't know what I am going to do when this happens and will probably be an incredible basket case when it does. So please have mercy and show compassion and give me all the affection you can even if you think I am overbearing because it will be so bad you will have to be willing to deal with it, I can't help it. If you are not willing to deal with it and still be compassionate you will probably cause me to lose my will to live. It is very important I sense your concern and interest to care how I feel. Thanks.

My mother wanted me to be taken care of after she dies. I especially need my wife to do all this for me. I will need everyone else in my life to do what they can to comfort me, the people at church, in the neighborhood, and nurses and doctors and techs in the medical community all need to be willing to give me comforting hugs.

The hospital staff and doctor's offices need to always give me "chipper acting, cheery female nurses" only, never male nurses or techs or serious trended female nurses or techs.

My nurses need to stick with me no matter what I say or do that annoys them or offends them. They need to be willing to accept all my idiosyncrasies and never judge me for what adults think and punish me for thinking kid thoughts because they interpret my kid needs, wants, and desires as being that of an adult's. They need to be wiling to forgive me for anything I say that offends them.

I need to receive lots of affection and attention from all my nurses, doctors, techs, friends, church friends, and neighbors at all times.

Brian Evans
49

I need to be treated like a person with special needs because that is who I am.

Not doing so traumatizes me to a great degree.

Have you ever seen the movie "Cipher in the Snow" where the kid is so downhearted that he asks to get off a bus one day on the way to school stating he needed to take a break and as soon as he stepped of the bus he fell into the snow and died? This is how severely not giving me hugs affects me.

The male lab techs at the military hospital that did blood tests on me made fun of me. They rammed needles in me and they laughed at me and thought it was funny. All the other doctors and nurses that did the shots were mean, stern, and gruff with me too.

The "serious trended female nurses" treated me like I was a piece of property to them and kicked me around like a dog, just like the men. Some of them even told me I was their property. It was very bad.

The "Chipper acting, cheery female nurses" always comforted me the way I wanted them to.

I never want a "male nurse" or "serious trended female nurse" in any hospital setting or doctor's office ever again. I was tortured by both of these the first several years of my life and both scare me

I also need lady friends to come visit me at my house every now and then and do girly things with me. Having guys over, especially after a death, would not be helpful to me. This will only depress me and make me feel even worse. This is especially true if they talk about doing guy stuff with me to pass the time. This is the last thing I need. I need lady friends to come and check on me and hug me, and comfort me, and make sure I am okay. I need them to act like mothers to me when this happens.

I need to be able to do girly stuff and kiddy stuff with them like have tea parties, watch kid movies, have a birthday party with them present or them visit while I color books or something. Maybe they can sit on the porch and have coffee with us and look at the flower garden or sit on the couch with us while we watch movies or color, or play games if I'm not too depressed to do so.

When I was in special Ed this is who I mainly stuck around was ladies, and it's even that way with Bingo too. I do have a couple of guy friends at Bingo, yes, but I talk to and associate with the ladies the most. That is who I am comfortable with and relate to the most.

This is what I need is the comfort and socialization of lady friends.

"Unpredictable changes and constant variations in day-to-day care upset a stressed patient and may throw him into panic."
   Using Crisis Intervention Wisely, Nursing Skillbook, page 42, Intermed Communications, Inc., 1979

I was in the hospital a few years ago; I had the perfect nurse for the day. She was so sweet and compassionate. She was always checking on me to see if I needed anything. This is exactly what I needed. She asked me if I wanted something to drink. I said, "Yes. Could you get me a soda, water and coffee?" She said she would be right back. Well, in walks someone else with my drinks! I was thrown into a full panic! I thought I did something wrong to make her mad I thought something was terribly wrong!

The charge nurses need to understand how important it is not to change nurses in the middle of the shift when the patient is comfortable with their nurse because it causes extra stress on the patient. If it is absolutely necessary the nurses need to be sure to explain the change to their patients.

Brian Evans

The nurses and nurse aids that take care of me that are asked to go to a different floor or ward in the middle of a shift also need to tell me before they leave that they were just asked to go to a different floor or ward by their charge nurse and that they will be back in a couple of hours or as soon as they can be when this happens so I will know there is nothing wrong I did to run them off. That way I don't have to worry constantly that I must have done something wrong to run them off because someone else walked in the room instead of them when they were the ones that were supposed to return with my stuff or return to check on me.

I get really freaked out over the craziest things even when nothing is wrong to begin with. I am very sensitive emotionally and get my feelings hurt very easily.

I care so much about what people think of me if I think someone doesn't like me I get scared. I worry constantly about offending my nurses I'm getting. This is a constant problem for me even if I've done nothing wrong worthy of punishment. I'm just strange that way, like someone that gets fidgety over things easily.

"Respect your patient's limitation. Don't expect too much from him, especially on days his routine has been upset."
>Using Crisis Intervention Wisely, Nursing Skillbook, page 42, Intermed Communications, Inc., 1979

Many people have failed to realize what my limitations are, my friends, and my bosses at places I worked as well as nurses who work with me. When they expect too much of me, I get overwhelmed.

When my bosses expected too much of me; I was not physically able to perform up to their expectations. I wound up becoming more severely ill as a result. As far as normalcy goes, various friends have misunderstood this in the past, but that is much better now.

"The trouble with denial and other psychologic defenses is, they interfere with your perception. When this happens, you leave your crisis patient without the support he needs to restore his equilibrium."

> Using Crisis Intervention Wisely, Nursing Skillbook, page 42, Intermed Communications, Inc., 1979

"You may see an occasional patient who hides extreme stress under an unusually calm, composed exterior. Try to estimate his internal stress level. It may be greater than that of the patient who shows distress."

> Using Crisis Intervention Wisely, Nursing Skillbook, page 42, Intermed Communications, Inc., 1979

"Whatever you do, never give a patient or his family the impression that you are criticizing them, trying to impart your own values or acting as their judge."

> Using Crisis Intervention Wisely, Nursing Skillbook, page 42, Intermed Communications, Inc., 1979

I have never responded well to criticism and always respond better to positive reinforcement. They were really good about this in Special Ed. The normal world just wanted to use constructive criticism. I felt like I could never meet up to anybody's standards again no matter what I tried. Because of this I felt like I was not good enough for anybody. I was even told this by some people. I do better when I don't feel like I am a complete failure to people. I don't want to always feel like I have to be hammered for everything by everybody all the time.

You never know when I might say something like a child. I often get misunderstood and criticized for what I say. I often say something not even thinking just like a kid would. Someone might respond with, "Did you realize what you just said?" I would be like "No." It's kind of like the disciple Peter that speaks before he thinks at times. I have the same problem. You just have to get around me a while to notice it.

"In recognizing the pre-combative patient, the best way to deal with combative behavior is to anticipate it and intervene before the situation gets out of control. Watch for unusual behavior that identifies the potentially combative patient. For instance, does he: seem elated, restless, agitated? Demand constant attention from everyone? Talk loudly or boisterously? Tease and bait others constantly with sarcasm? Pepper his conversation with vulgarities and profanities? Show a limited attention span? Remember, what the frustrated, angry patient needs most is not to suppress these troublesome feelings, but to free himself of them by expressing them. Help him do this if you can, while protecting him from hurting himself and others."

> Using Crisis Intervention Wisely, Nursing Skillbook, page 80, Intermed Communications, Inc., 1979

I've always demanded a lot of attention and affection and this is who I am and what I need. I actually require a lot of attention and affection to be able to function normally and feel mentally stable.

"If your patient's behavior suggests he may become combative: place someone in charge of decision making. If the patient has to be forcefully restrained, someone will have to decide when all other forms of intervention have failed. Choose someone who'll relate best to the patient to do the interacting. This might be his "favorite nurse", an aide, or doctor."

> Using Crisis Intervention Wisely, Nursing Skillbook, page 81, Intermed Communications, Inc., 1979

I've never been a combative patient as an adult before. As a child at the military hospital I was combative. Only because of the mean way I was treated by the "male" doctors, "male" nurses and techs, and "serious trended female" nurses. I almost never got a "chipper acting, cheery female" nurse. When I did, which was rare, they were a whole lot nicer. Things went a whole lot better and a whole lot smoother. They always acted nice, understood me, and met all my emotional needs and understood my pain, fear, anxiety, and differences, unlike the rest of the bunch.

The best way to ever handle a situation like this with me, if it ever did happen, is to get my favorite nurse. If my favorite nurses work with me to begin with it will probably prevent anything like this happening in the first place.

"You may have to restrain a patient long enough to give him a sedative. Use your weight to pin his torso and legs to the bed"
> Using Crisis Intervention Wisely, Nursing Skillbook, page 80, Intermed Communications, Inc., 1979

In the picture on this page, one nurse is leaning over with her arms spread over the patient's back. Another nurse is on his opposite side holding down one hip while she gives him the injection in the other hip. The other nurse has one of the legs bent at the knee with her hands holding his leg in place where it is bent in the underside of the knee.
> Using Crisis Intervention Wisely, Nursing Skillbook, page 80, Intermed Communications, Inc., 1979

"When you give an I.V. injection to a combative patient, brace his arm so he can't bend his elbow. Protect yourself by stooping beside bed."
> Using Crisis Intervention Wisely, Nursing Skillbook, page 81, Intermed Communications, Inc., 1979

In the picture on this page, one nurse is leaning on one side holding his arm down straight at the wrist while giving him an IV injection at the mid arm below the tourniquet. The other nurse is leaning over him on the opposite side of the bed with one hand on the side of his upper chest. Her other hand was on his lower stomach.

That is how this picture shows these two nurses restraining this patient to do an IV injection.
> Using Crisis Intervention Wisely, Nursing Skillbook, page 81, Intermed Communications, Inc., 1979

I have never had to have this done to me before regardless of any misunderstandings there may have been in the past.

Brian Evans

I think the only way you would have to worry about this with me is if you refused to meet my needs and took me by force. I need to have a chipper acting female nurse to rub my head to calm me down and hold my hand through the IV stick. My needs are genuine and they need to be met or I will walk leave.

This book has this to say about a patient that tries to get away.

"First, recognize that he's asking for help. Don't try to stop him physically. Instead, try to find out why he wants to leave. By doing so you divert his energy, and get him to focus on the immediate problem, which you may be able to remedy."
Using Crisis Intervention Wisely, Nursing Skillbook, page 81, Intermed Communications, Inc., 1979

If you insisted on treating me whether I liked it or not and refused to meet my comfort needs you would have to take me by force. It is my right to refuse medical care if I am not happy with the situation. Cordial acting female nurses will not work, even if they are willing to meet my needs. They need to be more than a person who is just acts nice that smiles, I can tell the difference. They need to have a natural bouncy, go getter personality. They need to be fun loving and adventurous like someone off a Disney movie. I'll give you some examples from a few movies I enjoy: Aerial on the Little Mermaid, Anastasia, Anna on Frozen, or Frauline Maria or Eliza Doolittle on My Fair Lady. I need to be treated with motherly love and compassion from my nurses. If my nurses would just treat me as if I were their own child we would be set as long as they brought me comfort the way I ask them to.

I had some really traumatizing experiences from Birth through my 20s in both the medical field and in a school setting. A bunch of nurses in the medical field did different things, which may be taken as graphic in nature to me.

I also have a situation where a different group of people think I'm the bad guy.

Brian Evans
56

A group of college girls thought I was some sort of freak based on body language I was taught to have by opera instructors for a play I was in. They wouldn't leave me alone about it since. Because of their false opinions of me based on my training I had I fear you will not believe me about the different things I claim all these doctors and nurses did to me in the medical field. Thanks to them, I feel like you sure won't believe me about what the mental health staff did to me at the institution from age 13 to age 14 ½ because they think I'm the bad guy.

 In case you think I am making this up I saw something on the news once where a movie star was criticized to no end over looking like whoever the bad guy was they played in some film they did, when they didn't even have the kind of personality in real life that the character they played would have. Try that for a big misunderstanding.

Even I got a big surprise about "Little House on the Prairie" when I saw a new thing on it where they interviewed the actors. Ready for this, Nellie Olson's brother is really Melissa Gilbert's brother, the one that played Willie.

The girl that played Nellie Olson didn't act anything like Nellie Olson in real life and she felt bad that she had to act mean to Melissa Gilbert in pretense because Melissa was playing Laura Ingalls because, ready for the big shock, Melissa Gilbert and the girl that played Nellie Olson are friends.

That girl felt very awkward having to act that way toward Melissa Gilbert because that was not her true personality. So, just as she felt awkward about it, I felt awkward about having to look the way I looked by pretending to be a navy soldier in a chorus of H.M.S. Pinafore.

As a result of having trouble getting the body language down until I finally got stuck that way, then I looked awkward to everyone else.

Brian Evans
57

After I did, I was continually harassed from that day forward for being something I was not.

Not only do I have a traumatic medical experience with male doctors, nurses, and techs and serious trended female nurses in the medical setting, but one year in college I had trouble with girls cutting me down over my body language I had learned off of a group of opera people that choreographed my body movements for this play I was in, H.M.S. Pinafore, years earlier, making them look odd. Because of this I was continually accused of sexual harassment, being a wife beater, a womanizer, prince charming that thought he was God's gift to women and continually slammed from every direction over it.

It wasn't because I said or did any inappropriate things that could have been taken wrong, or made any sexual advances toward anybody as they would try to make you think. I never did anything wrong to anybody.

It was because, I smiled the wrong way, I walked in the door the wrong way, I picked up the coffee pot the wrong way, I had a swelled jaw, I rose my shoulders up and pushed them back in a tense way, and walked like a beam pole and talked like an amplifier. All these were results of my training, and all these got me in trouble.

They also said that a man with a low voice was a villain.

My voice was low at the time but luckily the pitch of my voice has gone back up like it was when I was a kid now.

People react better to that. It felt kind of weird to have a voice in the rocks to express a heart that's in the clouds. It gave a false impression of me and caused everybody to think I was some captain type or soldier type or villain type when I'm not captain like, soldier like, or villain like at all.

I'm actually nothing but a little peon coward that whimpers over the least little thing that scares me.

I have certain timidness about me that most people don't realize I have. I'm also a sentimentalist. In some ways I can be really bold but in many other ways, I'm really shy.

People would probably notice if they paid more attention before they judged. But because having a voice that deep made me look like I was putting on a show, they said I was full of hot air when I wasn't even the way I looked at all.

They even said a man with bushy eyebrows is a villain and I have bushy eyebrows.

I found out later about that most autistic people have bushy eyebrows and I'm autistic.

Somebody out there was probably being prejudiced and just wanted to make false accusations about people that didn't make sense to them.

Just because you're different doesn't make you bad.

Have you ever seen the movie "Princes Diaries" and what they did to make her look different? Did you see how harshly her peers responded to her when they made her look different?

That's what they did to me. That's how they reacted to me. They reacted even worse toward me for the exact same reasons they did that girl. Because of this traumatic experience when someone gets the least little wrong idea about me I automatically think, "What if they think what they thought?"

I go way out on a rampage with it and people don't know what to think.

What's happening is I am putting these people's words in your mouth because of fear of what you will think of me.

I did that once after a male Director of Speech Pathology misunderstood why I wanted female therapist.

He thought I was after the women because I wouldn't take a guy for a therapist. He was very stern about it.

As a result, I thought, "Oh no! He reminds me of my 5th grade History teacher who tried to turn my 7th grade Special Ed English teacher against me! He might try to turn my favorite IV helper against me and all of his therapists!"

So, as a result, I wrote all of them trying to defend myself of this man.

I feared if he lied about me, they would begin to say, think and do what these college girls did to me over 20 years ago.

It's just an automatic panic response.

What they witnessed me doing was nothing other than a "panic attack". This was triggered by a present situation that I associated with a past situation that was similar in nature. I never did anything to anybody, nor was I going to. I just freaked out and panicked.

And that's why I wrote the letters, not because I was evil, but because I was having what's called a "panic attack".

It probably never occurred to this guy that women work better with Special Ed people than do men.

Because I haven't been in Special Ed since the 7th grade he probably couldn't tell I'd ever been in Special Ed so he probably thought I was normal.

He acted like he was too dumb to even figure out I even had a problem. He acted like he thought I was just pretending to have a disability because I sounded fine to him. Men can't usually tell right off, but most women can tell even when men cannot. Women are usually better at figuring out how to deal with disabled people. Women are also better at knowing how to meet their needs the right way especially if a person has a dependency problem like I do who needs motherly chipper acting females for his nurses and therapists.

Now, let's take this a step further.

I'm already worried you will believe what these girls thought of me based on my body language was true. Because of this, if I told you that "male doctors and nurses and techs" tortured me with needles and demanded I undress myself in front of them at the military hospital you might not believe me. And if I told you the "serious trended female nurses" also tortured me with needles, ripped my clothes off of me, and threw a gown on me when I refused to cooperate with them, after you already have preconceived ideas about me based on what these college girls thought of me because of my opera training, there's no telling what you might think of me.

My next thought is going to be, "Oh no! Now they're really going to think I'm weird because these college girls thought I was some sort of sex fiend when all I did was walk, talk, and act like some royal person out of the 1800s and when they hear that these people at the military hospital did this to me, they're going to think I'm making all this up and really think they have to worry about me when there's nothing to worry about to begin with."

Then, if I told you two men and a stern woman constantly made me take my clothes off in front of a room full of boys at a mental institution from June 1, 1982 to October 24, 1983 to punish me for being different in hopes to humiliate me, you're horrible thoughts of me are heightening.

"I knew he was perverted! Look at this! He's making up inappropriate stories about naked people!"

Then if I told you that in April 1983 a slim, slightly broad shouldered chipper acting, cheery female staff lady with shoulder length brown hair protected against the blonde heavy set guy that was doing this to me and she was the lady I rubbed the feet of, you would probably think, "I wonder what's going on with that! Does he have something going with this lady?!"

Even though you're probably not paying attention, I am telling you this guy was looking at me from the other side of the room wishing he could find a way to punish me. He wanted to make me take my clothes off in front of a room full of boys to humiliate me but he was afraid to do this to me in front of her because she might not approve of what he was doing if he tried.

Because of how judgmental people have responded to me before when I tell them things like this I figured you would probably think, "I knew it! He's talking about naked people again! How dare he talk this kind of nonsense to us! Who does he think he is?!"

So then if I told you that when I sat with this lady on the couch, I thought, "Hah! I'm safe with this lady! He won't make me take my clothes off in front of everybody when she's around!" I fear you will think, "I knew it! He's talking sexual again! He said something about this man making him take his clothes off when this lady is around!"

If I told you this lady was my "protection" against this blonde heavy set guy while she worked there and after she was gone two months later I suddenly felt like I had to see every lady's and girl's feet and toes everywhere for the first time ever from that day forward, you might think, "I knew it! He has a foot fetish too! Who does he think he is? Is he after us or something?"

Brian Evans
62

Now, to make it worse, suppose you are my nurse and you think I am a horrible person based on all these terrible things I've told you and I have to show you a rash I got that month that had to be taken care of. As a result you had to see something private in order to take care of it.

Now you're thinking, "Now he's really done it! How dare he ask me to look at a rash?! There better be a rash there! He better not be pulling the flax over my eyes! This is totally inappropriate and totally unacceptable!"

You think you have a case now.

These girls thought all this horrible stuff about me at a college over 20 years ago that wasn't true. I've told you what they did to me at the military hospital and the institute that was graphic in nature. Then, out of nowhere I came down with a rash and you think I've really done it now.

All this horrible chaos is going through my mind over what you will think of me if you know all these things. Now it's troubling me and sending me into high stress which could throw me into a crisis situation when my fears are escalated that I may be misjudged.

As a result, when I react in panic, you act in haste because you think I am the bad guy and want to punish the living daylights out of me.

I've actually been frightened for a long time that this will happen and you will think all of these things about me.

Sometimes I feel like I'm about to panic because of all this.

This is why I will probably get all freaked out. If I'm not sure what you are thinking about me and fear you may not know what to make of my odd needs and odd behaviors I'm scared to death you'll do the opposite of what I need because of this.

Brian Evans

You may even jump down my throat about something that isn't even true just because it appears true to you. So, now you're mad for sure and you want to let me have it because you think I am the most horrible person you ever saw based on your misjudgment of what is happening here.

I just want you to see who the real Brian Evans is and what the real Brian Evans needs. I need you to see me as an autistic individual that used to be in Special Ed that was normalized into looking like something he's not and treat him like the special needs person he really is. I need you to treat me like a Special Ed person again like people did before this whole thing ever happened and meet my special needs. Please see to it that you do this for me.

If anyone does not believe my stories about what happened at the institution or the military hospital my mother knows they did it.

She has some memory problems because of old age, but when she's having a good day and can remember everything well enough to get things straight she can tell you I am telling you the truth about all this happening.

She also knows about the girls at the college.

She also knows the truth about what happened at the institution and the military hospital.

Most of the terrible experiences I had at the military hospital took place between Birth and age 15. The rest took place between age 16 and 21. This took place from March 3, 1969 to July 1990.

The bad experiences at the mental institution took place between age 13 and 14 ½. This took place from June 1, 1982 to October 24, 1983.

My mother knows what happened in all of these instances. She knows I'm telling the truth about the shirt tail punishments at the mental institution I was in for a year and a half.

Brian Evans
64

She knows that means these people put me on display for other people to look at in only my underwear and a white undershirt with colored sleeves.

She knows I was tortured with needles by the "male doctors", "male nurses", and "serious trended female nurses" at the military hospital.

She knows the "chipper acting, cheery female nurses" always understood me. She knows they did well with me and met my needs the way I needed them met in a cheerful way. She knows they were much more understanding and much more productive with me when I did get them.

She also knows that unfortunately, it was very rare for me to ever receive a chipper acting female nurse at the military hospital and only got that lucky in two or three isolated instances.

Almost every time it was a "male nurse".

And, the times it was not a "male nurse", it was almost always a "serious trended female nurse" with a cranky personality who acted almost as bad as the men and were very forceful and demanding themselves. These ladies were also "down your throatish" in the way they asked you to do things. These were "straight faced" ladies that never got excited about anything and never smiled.

The Radiology Techs and ER Techs weren't any better.

We're talking about a military hospital here.

Think about that one for a minute. You can get some mean doctors and nurses in a setting like that.

Also, think about this one. The one mean woman I got at the mental institution from age 13 to 14 ½ was an ex-army cadet. She bragged about this like she thought it made her powerful.

Brian Evans
65

Take that in account when you think about how she might have treated me when she demanded I take my clothes off in front of a room full of boys.

This happened several times at the institution I was in.

Sounds scary doesn't it?

Do you still want to judge me for being inappropriate because I said a woman did this to me? Now you know "what kind" of woman did this to me? That's why.

My mother did not know specifically that these "serious trended" female nurses at the military hospital forcibly stripped me when they took me to a room to torture me with needles because she wasn't there to see it. They made her stay in the lobby.

When I asked her if she remembered being asked to sit in a lobby by the first doctor I saw while these two ladies took me down a hall to another room to do the rest of the patient care, she said she thought she did vaguely remember that.

When I asked her, "Is it my imagination or do you think these "serious trended female nurses" actually stripped me of my clothes and shoved the hospital gown on me when they took me to a room to examine me and torture me with needles? I keep seeing these scenes in my mind of two disgruntled female nurses taking me down a hall to a room. After they took me in the room, one of them got in my face yelling at me. I was scared and backed up toward the door trying to escape. They were yelling, "Is there a problem?! Is there a problem?! Is there some kind of problem?! Do you want to be a problem?! Are you going to change into your gown or are we going to do it for you?! Take his clothes off and put the gown on him!" She grabbed me by the wrists and pushed me against the wall while the other one jerked my clothes off and shoved the gown over my chest. Then, they drug me to a bed, practically threw me on it, and proceeded to ram needles in me as hard as they could.

Brian Evans
66

Do you think this really happened, or I'm I just imagining all this?"

She said, "I wouldn't put it past them. If you think you remember them doing something like this, they probably did."

And, I thought, "That's what I thought. So, it's not my imagination. This really did happen."

"I also remember these "serious trended female nurses" threatening me when they proceeded to come after me with a needle yelling, "You think you're scared of us now! You're really going to be scared of us when we're done with you! If you don't stop screaming I'm going to make her stick you again! Stick him again! Stick him again!"

Like I said, these nurses "were not" chipper acting nurses, they were "serious trended female nurses".

They were nothing but a bunch of straight faced, cranky, domineering, forceful, tyrannical, disgruntled, military women that wanted to shift their weight around and demand cooperation or force it on you.

I think the male doctors and nurses also tackled me and pinned me down a lot to do what they did because they were so rough I'd try to resist them and they would force me to cooperate with them.

I don't remember the men stripping me down but they may have.

I do remember these "male doctors" and "male nurses" demanding I take my clothes off in front of them. They would sternly say, "Get undressed! You need to put on this gown!" I was so scared of them I just did what they said. I figured if I didn't do what they said they would have forcibly stripped me like the "serious trended female nurses" did. They were that mean. They were not about to take "no" for an answer. They made it clear I was going to do what they said or else.

Brian Evans

Also, when I went to the lab techs to get my blood drawn they had big fat, marinade tubes with big long fat needles that scared me to death.

I was scared and they would make fun of me and say, "Do we have a baby in here? Do we have a baby in here? I think we have a baby in here!"

Screaming in pain, I would say, "Do you have very far left to go? Are you almost done yet?"

They bragged and said, "No! We have a long way to go!" as they filled the thing full so they could fill several tubes of blood to make my life miserable and laugh about it while they did it.

Then they would say, "Boy, this guy's having trouble here! We need to make a man out of this guy! Maybe you'll do better the next time!" laughing as they said it.

These men also rammed their needles in me and had a blast doing it and loved it that I was scared of them and the needle.

When I went to the male ER techs on several occasions, they acted more gruff like the male doctors and nurses did I saw and yelled at me like they did, rammed needles in me like they did, and got rough with me and said condescending things to me like they did and forced my every move.

I wonder if that male Director of Speech Pathology I told you about would see why I wanted a female therapist now if he knew what happened with these men. That might be enlightening on his part. He should have thought about that when I asked him for a female therapist. I always had trouble with male everything and that's why I wanted a female because they are more compassionate and understand me better. I was never after anyone. I just didn't want men because of how I was treated by men in the past. I met this Director of Speech Pathology two decades after the worst of all this occurred.

Brian Evans

I just want you to see why I felt the way I did when he judged me. It would have been about a decade and a half after the last time I went to the military hospital.

My mother knows these men did this to me. She saw them do it.

If you called my mother, she could tell you I am telling the truth. She knows I do not have the tendency to lie.

She knows I always doing everything I can to make sure I tell the truth about everything no matter how far fetched it may sound.

The only problem is she is having memory problems now due to old age. She may not always remember everything at the spur of the moment until it comes back to her. This may vary from day to day.

If you didn't believe me about this you could always ask her if she happens to remember at the time you call her what happened.

You would just have to hope it was a day she was having a good memory if you did and then she could tell you I'm telling the truth.

If you nurses wonder why in the world I would get such outlandish ideas about what you would think about everything I ever say it is because when I lived in Abilene, Texas I ran into a lot of judgmental people that were really bad about thinking these kinds of thoughts toward me. I felt like I couldn't say anything without them getting stirred up the wrong way. When I moved to Arkansas that all changed. People treated me normal again and didn't get all these weird ideas.

The only problem is, in a few situations where I just asked for my needs for comfort to be met by the nurses some hospitals and a few doctor's offices acted outraged that I would ask such horrible requests. They took the things I asked them to do that I desperately needed from them and made something horrible out of it that wasn't even there.

Brian Evans
69

ll I did was ask them for the hugs I needed, the chipper acting cheery female nurses, and the head rubs and hand holds through needle sticks I needed by these chipper acting cheery female nurses with motherly personalities.

They just judged me based on what they thought everyone else looked like and acted like and thought to themselves, "If a normal person would have asked me to do these things for them they would have thought this horrible thing or that horrible thing."

If they would have just taken me for my word to begin with things would have been a lot better. They should have seen the situation for what it is.

I am autistic and have childlike needs that need to be met by my nurses and always have had these needs my entire life.

It would have solved the whole problem and everything would have gone a whole lot smoother if they had just given in and met them freely.

I had a hospital that did this for me for 10 years straight. The problem is they had a major turnover in nurses and all the nurses I had that ever understood me quit their jobs.

They hired all new ones that were stoic to take their place that were only there for the check.

That's why I came to you. So you could treat me like they did before everything went sour.

In my heart I feel like you probably will not think these terrible things I fear you might think about me that I just told you about.

However, because of these past experiences with being judged wrongly for all this, I feel like I need a few experiences with you in each department of your hospital that go well where you understand me and meet my needs first before I can have total reassurance you will not think this way or feel this way about me.

Plus, it will help me a great deal, if you let me know verbally that you believe me about what I say happened and you do not think any of this horrible stuff about me or have to worry that I will.

I also have this fear that if I ever should need assistance in the hospital setting with bathing, toileting, or changing gowns that you as my female nurses will throw me off on a guy because you don't want bothered with it. I don't want a male nurse for anything. I want the chipper acting, cheery female nurses for everything even if it means having to do private things like this.

I'm also afraid if I tell a nurse I have swelled ankles or a white patch at the bottom of my leg where hair disappeared or have a rash that needs checked I ask them to look at that they will think I am being inappropriate, when I am in fact being serious.

I'm not going to tell you there is something wrong when there's not anything wrong. If I tell you something is wrong you can count it on that what I am saying is true.

Please don't think of me as an adult male when you have to do this but think of me as a baby in diapers when you have to do these kinds of things for me. Thanks.

Now let's take all this and reevaluate this thing.

There are things in all these stories that gave it away that none of the terrible things you are thinking about me are true.

First, why did the girls at the college think I was some kind of perverted freak in the first place? Was it because I said or did anything wrong? No.

Brian Evans
71

Did I make any sexual advances toward anyone or do anything inappropriate toward them? No.

What was the reason for the whole thing?

I was trained by a bunch of opera people for a play years earlier that made me smile with my teeth, pull my shoulders back and lock them into place, walk like a beam pole, talk like an amplifier, pick up a coffee pot like a robot, open door knobs like bank vault latches, lock my jaw in a certain way to produce certain musical sounds that made my jaw tight and eventually swelled.

And, I was only out of Special Ed for 3 years before I was even trained for this play.

How do you think being trained to look like some royal person from the 1800s and getting stuck looking like that because your trainers thought you would never get it right and when you finally did it you got stuck that way and people didn't know what to think is going to look on you?

They also made me think and analyze things in a way a rich person would when I was nothing but a peon. This didn't look right on me anyway because it looks awkward and doesn't make sense.

I've tried to make sense of an upper-class language I can never completely understand.

So, I wind up combining my Special Ed vocabulary with rich people's vocabulary and trying to make something out of it. I only catch pieces of what it all means to begin with and look really strange as a result. I don't know what's going on anymore. I don't know how to look anymore. I look somewhere half way between a rich person and a nearly retarded person.

And now, suddenly I now have a jagged intelligence because part of me gets their communication system and part of me doesn't so it all gets mixed.

Brian Evans
72

People don't know what to make of it, an intelligent looking person who looks awkward and says awkward things that they don't know used to be a Special Ed person that thought and acted like Special Ed people.

And now I think and act a little like both so now it's all mixed up and it has totally messed up my intelligence where it is no longer straight across.

It's not one way or the other anymore.

So now, people think I am extremely eccentric because of what I look like. My autism already makes me look odd to some extent by itself which I didn't know I had till over a decade after these people thought all this horrible stuff about me. And now because of my opera training I really look weird. When those opera people took someone like me that just looked a little odd and then trained me to look like them then it made me look really odd. That's why these girls reacted the horrible way they did to me. They never saw anything like this before and it didn't make sense to them.

What do you think is going to happen if you take an Ex-Special Ed person with their Special Ed mannerisms and mix their mannerisms with your rich upper-class mannerisms?

People try to make my new learned mannerisms which looks odd on me determine what my personality is.

They don't' know what to make of it. They try to compare it to what the normal everyday person looks like and here's what they think. What do normal everyday modern people look like when they act like this or look like this? "Oh, he must be a freak! This doesn't match our body language system or our communication system! Sexual Harassment!" just like they did to the girl on the "Princess Diaries" movie.

They didn't know what to make of her, so she must be freaky too. So now, I'm condemned for life.

Brian Evans
73

I feel like I always have to try to prove I am not what people think I am because "these people made me look like this".

What these people thought about me is the joke of the century. Bertha can tell you, I'm not a very sexual person. These people would feel really stupid if they figured that out.

No one ever really had anything to worry about because there was nothing to worry about. I'm not the bad guy they think I am.

Most mentally disabled people are not very sexual people. I've found that out through research when Bertha was looking up stuff on Autism. I found this out when we first found out I was autistic. Most of the stuff we read pointed out this very thing. Mentally disabled people really aren't very sexual in comparison to the normal every day person. Their drive is usually very low, and sometimes none at all. Mine is low. I am quite the opposite of what these girls I went to college with think. I was just trained to look like something else these girls didn't understand. My body language looked different from the norm as a result. They jumped on it. And, as a result, they jumped to conclusions in the process and we're wrong about the whole thing.

If I would have never found out I had the voice talent this would have never happened.

Something miraculous happened to my voice one day when I was 17. I was set up with a private voice instructor who trained me that wanted me to go to college. I thought he was crazy because I didn't think I'd ever make it. He changed his mind when a friend of his told him I was retarded. My mother was upset and said, "I don't care! I'm sending you anyway! If he thinks you can make it, you're going!"

As a result, all this stuff I'm telling you about is what happened. If I hadn't have gone it would have never happened but because I did, it did happen. I wish I'd never known.

Then everyone would know who I really was and I would not have all this over my head to ruin my reputation. No one ever thought I was a creep before I found out I had the voice. I'm not you. I'm an ex-Special Ed student that got thrown into regular classes in the 8th grade. If only people could see that, I wouldn't have this problem.

My mother also knows all about what happened with this. She thinks the whole thing is ridiculous. Most of my friends who know these girls acted this way also think this is ridiculous. This was an Abilene, Texas thing. No one ever acted this way about me up here.

Before I met my opera trainers no one acted that way about me down there either until these people messed up my body language.

Now for the second thing, "Male" nurses, "male" doctors and "male" techs really did torture me with needles at the military hospital. At times they did sternly demand I get undressed in front of them and put my hospital gown on before they proceeded to torture me with needles. They still tortured me with needles even when I was dressed. It just made them feel more powerful over me when they did make me undress in front of them so they did it for spite to get back at me for being so hard to deal with.

As a result, they felt like this gave them more control over me. These men felt like the more they stuck me with needles, the more trouble they had.

So, as a result, they thought, "See if he gets away from us if we make him take his clothes off first!" They did this to me to put me at their mercy. They were out for a power grab and this made them really happy because it made them feel like they were able to get me back for being difficult.

These military doctors and nurses and techs weren't nice like you are in Arkansas where you nicely, courteously, politely ask me to change into a gown. They talked to me like I'd better do what they say or they would take me by force.

Brian Evans

They did this to me when I hadn't even done anything to them worthy of punishment.

They were just trying to be mean.

The "serious trended" female nurses at the military hospital really did forcibly strip me of my clothes when I refused to cooperate with them. They were very demanding. Two of them would gang up on me at a time.

One would grab my wrists and drag me across the room and restrain me while another one stripped me down. The nurse that stripped me would force the gown over my chest, throw me on a patient bed and come after me with needles, just like the men did. And like the men, they would ram their needles in me as hard as they could and griped about it when I screamed. They were not very nice at all.

My greatest fear is that if you're hospital has almost all nice nurses in it, which I need, and I tell you all this happened in my past you will think, "That kind of thing never happens! Who does he think he is, suggesting anybody ever does anything like this anywhere? We've never heard of such a thing! No nurse has ever forcibly stripped a patient of their clothes against their will here! He has to be making this up! No nurse has ever forcibly stripped any patient of their clothes anywhere or we would have known about it!"

Actually, think again.

Chances are you are right. If you are one of these especially nice hospitals with all nice nurses who care about the patient's dignity, there probably isn't any nurse at your hospital that would do this. But, that doesn't mean they wouldn't do this somewhere else. That's what I'm getting at. If the place I'm going now is as nice as I think it is, I highly doubt anything like that ever happens there or ever will happen there.

I just want them to know that there are people in another places have done this, and I don't want to be accused of being perverted because I said someone else somewhere else did.

I don't know of any proof of any medical hospitals from research that have done this outside of my experiences with the military hospital and the institution I went to but have any of you ever heard of the book "A Force For Good"?

This lady said that her "serious trended" female nurses did the very thing to her I'm telling you they did to me at that military hospital. This lady's experience was at a mental institution, but still. Her "serious trended" female nurses told her to take off her clothes and step in a room sized bathtub naked in front of several other female patients who also stepped in the tub naked at the same time. The lady refused and when she did they told her if she refused to take her clothes off they would do it for her. When she still refused, these mean acting "serious trended" female nurses grabbed the lady patient and forcibly stripped her of all her clothes against her will and forced her to step in the bath tub and bathed her against her will. I think I read these "serious trended" female nurses even got rough with her in the bathtub.

If you don't believe me about this, look it up on the Internet and see for yourself. It's on there. There was actually a court case about this incident at this institution because it really happened.

Have you ever seen the movie, "Girl Interrupted"?

This is a true story movie about a girl that mental health staff did the very things to I am telling you they did to me.

This girl aggravated the "serious trended" female staff at the institution she was in by her behavior patterns they didn't like. When they got fed up, they drug her down a hall and forcibly stripped her of all her clothes and threw a hospital gown on and made her run around barefooted in a hospital gown in front of everybody for probably a week.

Brian Evans
77

They had already done this to the blonde girl that was a troublemaker who gave this girl trouble and made her run around barefoot in a hospital gown in front of everybody in the lobby that was connected to the kitchen while all the other patients got to eat their food in the kitchen fully dressed and saw her undressed. This was a true story movie.

I even saw about 5 true story movies about mental institutions for boys and 2 true story movies about mental institutions for girls when I was about 15 years old, one year after I got out of the institution I was in.

In almost every one of these movies, they actually showed the patient getting in an argument with the nurses. The patient would run down a long hall in the building and the nurses would be chasing them. Then, about 3/4ths of the way down the hall, they would grab them in a doorway and shove them into the sidewall, and four different nurses, both men and women would be restraining this guy while they squirmed around and one of them would actually start pulling their pants off while another one got a hold of their shirt and jerked it off their chest and another nurse would pull their shoes and socks off while the other nurse held them against the sidewall next to the door. Then, another nurse would grab a hospital gown and proceed to shove it over their chest, opened the door and then shoved them in a room and locked them in there. They didn't care if anyone else was standing around watching either. They did this right in front of everybody.

I don't think there were any other patients hanging around in the hall in this movie when this happened, but I've seen movies where there were several other people around and they actually stripped these people down right in front of everybody.

I even saw them do this to their patients and then force them to wear hospital gowns in the kitchen area to eat while everyone else got to keep all their clothes on. They also made them stay like that in their living room lobbies while every one is was fully dressed.

That's what they did to these people and that's what they did to me. Only with me, in the institution, they gave me a choice. They demanded I take my clothes off in front of everybody in the room. I obediently did what they said, and after I took my shirt, and my pants, and my shoes and socks off right in front of everybody as they demanded, they handed me a white undershirt with colored sleeves and said, "Put this on!" Had I refused to do what they said, they would have tackled me down and stripped me down themselves.

Now, at the military hospital, that really was a forcible stripping, but this was a demand to undress myself at the institute, and would have resulted in a forcible stripping had I refused to do what they said.

I'm trying to tell you, I'm not lying.

Most chipper acting female nurses would never do something like this to somebody, but a "serious trended" female nurse would.

And, again, if you don't believe me, ask my mother, she knows the whole thing because all this stuff I'm telling you about happened when I was a kid.

When I tell you I fear a "serious trended" female nurse will do this to me as an adult, no it has never happened to me as an adult, but I have run into some very forceful nurses that were "serious trended" females that tried to force my every move at a couple of places. They also tortured me with needles as hard as they could and even jerked a catheter around in me and refused to comfort me. That's pretty bad.

What you have to think about is this; I was already changed into a hospital gown at the request of a "chipper acting, cheery female nurse in another department that never acted this way toward me before I went to these bad people.

So, let's reevaluate this situation, and ask the following question, "What would have happened if I hadn't already changed into a hospital gown for a "chipper acting, cheery female nurse" in a different department and I ran into these people and they made it obvious they were going to manhandle me from the start?

What would they have done if I would have refused to change into a hospital gown for them because I was afraid they would manhandle me?"

You get the picture. You see what I mean now.

What else do you think their going to do? Knowing people with their personality, their probably going to get mad and strip me down and force me to cooperate with them. That's what happened at the military hospital and that's what happened at the institution. I'm actually worried sick you'll refuse to give me a "chipper acting, cheery female nurse" because I said that these "serious trended female" nurses that acted "worse than the wicked witch of the west" forcibly stripped me of my clothes.

In your mind, you're thinking, "He said a woman did this. I'm not about to give him a female nurse if this is the case. He might be perverted."

Think about what I just said. That's like saying because he said the "Wicked Witch of the West" did this to him I'm not about to give him Dorothy.

If you think about it The Wicked Witch of the West obviously has a different personality than Dorothy. They are nothing alike.

Instead of protecting Dorothy from me because of what I said the Wicked Witch of the West did to me, you need to protect me by giving me Dorothy instead of the Wicked Witch of the West.

If you really think about it she was mean to Dorothy too.

Brian Evans
80

Don't think, "Oh! A woman! I knew there was something wrong here!"

What you need to think is, "What kind of woman did this?

A woman that acts like a witch and wants to control their patients and treat them like some piece of property they can kick around and do whatever they feel like to them and force their every move no matter what that means or a woman who is sweet and kind, and loving, and compassionate, and caring, and loving, and huggable, and encourageable and comforting and understanding?

The answer to that one is obvious. It would be the one that saw their patients as a piece of property they could just kick around and do whatever they felt like to them and force their every move. It sure wouldn't be the second one.

I will not be refused a "chipper acting, cheery female nurse" because of what I said a "witchy acting serious trended female nurse" did. That's why they did it, because they were a witch and the "chipper acting cheery female nurse" wasn't.

Have you ever seen the movie "Samantha" from American girl?

These ladies acted similar to the grumpy lady at the orphanage, only worse.

You wouldn't refuse to give me Samantha or Nellie Omallie, or Bridgette, or Jenny because of what I said the grumpy lady at the orphanage. Mrs. Fraucie did to me would you?

If I told you Cinderella's stepmother did this to me you wouldn't refuse to give me Cinderella would you?

 If I said the witch that gave Snow White an apple did this to me you wouldn't refuse to give me Snow White would you?

If I said Rapunzel's stepmother on the movie "Tangled" did this to me would you refuse to give me Rapunzel?

If I said, Mrs. Carp did this to me on the movie "The Princess and the Pauper" would you refuse to give me Erica or Analise?

If I said Ursula did this to me on the movie "The Little Mermaid" would you refuse to give me Ariel?

Do you see what I'm getting at?

These are opposite personalities.

If I say that these mean women did what they did then they did what they did and their opposite would never do something like what they did then their opposite would be what I needed.

These women are the direct opposite of what I'm asking for.
I'm asking for a "chipper acting, cheery female nurse" who will be nice to me and understand me and comfort me the way I need comforted that will be there for me when I need them and help me.

I shouldn't be punished by not being given a female nurse at all, if I'm going to tell you that an evil acting one did something terrible to me, because the chipper ones are the ones I need and they have always been nice to me and met my needs happily.

Anytime I've told a "chipper acting female nurse" how a mean acting female nurse treated me in Arkansas if they knew them they would be like "Is that who you are afraid of? They scare me too."

Chances are, if these "chipper acting female nurses" saw the very individuals that did this to me at the military hospital and the institution in Abilene, Texas and saw how they acted they would not even like them. They would probably be afraid of them themselves.

Chances are if they saw who these people are I'm talking about they would probably say, "Is this the people that did this to you?" and I said, "Yes" they would probably say, "No wonder you were afraid of these people. I'm afraid of them too."

Chances are, if a mean nurse of that nature ever got a hold of me at a hospital up here, which has happened before, and a chipper acting, cheery female nurse caught these "serious trended" female nurses in the act of being mean to me and trying to torture me they would probably get irate with them and say, "Hey, Leave him alone! Pick on somebody your own size! He can't defend himself!" Then, if there was any way in the world possible they could do this for me, if they didn't feel like they had their hands tied by their boss, they would probably try to come to the rescue and say, "I'm so sorry that nurse was so mean to you. It's okay. I'll take care of you. You won't have to worry about that woman. That lady's mean. We've had problems with her being ugly to her patients before. But, you're safe now because I'm going to be your nurse. You just stick with me and you'll be okay. You let me know if you need anything. If you get scared I'm right here and I'll do whatever you need me to to help you. Don't worry about that other crazy woman. She's just mean."

Do you see what I mean now?

This is the kind of women I'm talking about that did this to me.

It was the cranky ones that act like the bad guys on all these movies that did this to me.

The ones that act all sweet like Dorothy, Samantha, Nellie Omallie, Bridgette, Jenny, Cinderella, Snow White, Rapunzel, Erica, Analise, and Ariel in the above examples were always nice to me and always good to me and comforted me and consoled me in the way I needed comforted and consoled.

It was the ones that act like the Wicked Witch of the West, Mrs. Fraucie who owned the orphanage, Cinderella's stepmother, the Evil Queen on Snow White, the Evil Stepmother on Rapunzel, Mrs. Carp on the "Princess and the Pauper" movie, and Ursula on the movie "The Little Mermaid" that acted this way toward me. They were the ones that forcibly stripped me of my clothes and tortured me with needles. Not the nice ones.

The nice ones were always good to me. They never approved of what these other personality types of nurses did to me. They were on my side and they loved me and always did everything they could to help me in the way I needed to when I got them.

If they ever knew something like this was going on, they would try to protect me from people like this.

So if I say someone that acted like the Wicked Witch of the West, Mrs. Fraucie, Cinderella's stepmother, the Evil Queen on Snow White, the Evil Stepmother on Rapunzel, Mrs. Carp on the "Princess and the Pauper" or Ursula forcibly stripped me of my clothes and tortured me with needles, don't refuse to give me someone that acts like Dorothy or Samantha or Nellie Omallie or Bridgette, or Jenny, or Cinderella, or Snow White, or Rapunzel, or Erica, or Analise, or Ariel, the little mermaid. That's who I need.

They are the ones I want to work with me, not these witchy people.

And, don't give me a man because I said some witchy acting woman forcibly stripped me of my clothes.

Just because I said a woman did this doesn't mean I'm perverted.

It means that a mean acting, controlling woman with a dictatorial personality that wants to make slaves out of their patients did this to me and that is why I am better off with the sweet, compassionate, friendly acting ones I am asking for.

So, please, don't refuse to give me who I'm asking for and who I need because of this.

The ones I'm asking for are completely the opposite personality of the ones that did this to me, and they're the ones I expect to get.

And, if you don't believe the "serious trended" female nurses did this to me and the "male doctors and nurses" did this to me, ask my mother. She knows. She was there.

Now, to really drive the point home, "Would you have refused to give me that nice brown haired lady that protected me from that man at the institution if I told you that red headed lady also demanded I take my clothes off in front of a room full of boys?"

That red headed lady did the same thing that blonde headed man did, and so did his black haired partner.

They all three did this to me. They took turns doing this to punish me by humiliating me for being different so they could make me what they wanted to be instead of accepting me for who I was. All of them did this, but this one chipper acting, cheery female staff person did not. The points about them are coming up after I tell you about the men at the military hospital. Be ready to read about it. You'll be enlightened as to what I went through.

Now you know what kind of people did this to me and who didn't.

Do you want to know why "male nurses" and "serious trended" female nurses forcibly strip their patients of their clothes in the medical hospital setting when it does happen?

The nurses that do this can't stand it that their patient is a coward. They don't want to have to put up with their squeamishness and squirminess and high strung fears of what they will do to them, even though they intend on doing the very things the patient fears they will do to them because they are that mean.

So, when they forcibly strip a patient of their clothes, they do it to "force cooperation" from their patient. They figure once they get their clothes off of them they can do anything they want to their patients no matter how much they fight them or try to resist them and there's not a thing they can do to stop them. So, then when they do begin to torture them with needles and yell and scream at them they are able to do so with full force. And, the patient who would like to get away from them if he could get away from them will be caught stark naked in front of everybody embarrassed to death if he even dares to try to get away from them and make a run for it. So, as a result, they have full control and they win in the end by evil means.

I found these two things recently through research.

"Dorothea Dix played an instrumental role in the founding of more than 30 hospitals for treatment of the mentally ill. She was a leading figure in those national and international movements that challenged the idea that people with mental disturbances could not be cured or helped. She also was a staunch critic of "cruel and neglectful practices toward the mentally ill", such as "caging", "incarceration without clothing", and "painful physical restraint".
> Dorothea Dix (1802-1887), Promoting Public Health
> Research Policy, Practice and Education, American Journal
> of Public Heath 2006

"Dorothea Dix may have had personal experience of mental instability that drove her to focus on the issue of asylum reform, and certainly her singular focus on the issue led to some important victories."
> Dorothea Dix (1802-1887), Promoting Public Health
> Research Policy, Practice and Education, American Journal
> of Public Heath 2006

Notice she said they "incarcerated their patients without clothing".

Hopefully, it's obvious what happened here.

I wanted to let you know the patients didn't just walk in there naked with no clothes on and these people find them and lock them up. That's not what happened here. I can tell you that right now from my own personal experience.

I can tell you right now, these patients that went in these asylums when into the asylum with all their clothes on.

What happened was, these patients were fully clothed when they walked in these places, but these people that took over their care forcibly stripped them of all their clothes and locked them up with no clothes on.

I know how it works. That's exactly what they did.

They did this to break their spirit and put them on public display for everyone to look at with no clothes on to embarrass the living daylights out of them and make them feel lower than low.

Their caretakers wanted to be in charge of them and they felt like if they stripped them of all their clothes they could do anything they wanted to do to them or make them do anything they wanted them to do and they would not be able to stop them because they would feel defenseless and intimidated and humiliated in front of them and feel inferior to their position above them as a staff member of that institution.

They did this to make them feel like they had no hope and they were there to stay as a slave to the ones that were over them and there was nothing they could do to change it. They were basically had and they knew it and they were nothing but a piece of property to these people and felt like helpless peons that couldn't do a thing about it. They treated them like they were their slaves. They felt like they were nothing but slaves and could not escape them.

In the book "Someone Else's Kids" by Tory Hayden, she has a story about the mother of an autistic boy that attends her Special Ed class.

In this story the mother tells all her concerns about what will happen to her boy because of his disability. She begins talking about an asylum she had visited that had a boy in it her husband knew and they were not nice to him either.

Here is what she has to say about this.

Mrs. Franklin said, "I don't want them to take him away," she interrupted still looking down at her hands. "I don't want them to put him in no insane asylum. I don't want them to take my boy away."

Tory said, "I can't imagine anyone will, Mrs. Franklin."

Mrs. Franklin said, "Charles, that's my husband, he says so sometimes. He says if Boothe Birney doesn't learn to talk straight like other boys, they're going to lock him away in an insane asylum when he grows up and we can't take care of him no more. Charles, he knows those things. He says Boothe Birney's sick and they don't let sick boys stay with their folks."

Tory said, "Boo isn't sick. He's just different."

Mrs. Franklin said, "Charles said they're going to take him away. The doctors, they'll do it. They told Charles. If Boothe don't learn to talk straight."

Tory said, "I found Mrs. Franklin difficult to reason with. She was so frightened."

Mrs. Franklin said, "They ain't good places, miss, them insane asylums. I seen one. My mother's brother they put him in one once in Arkansas. And I seen it."

Tory said, "She paused and the silence stabbed through me."

Mrs. Franklin said, "There was this big boy there," she said softly." "A great big boy, 'most nearly a man with yellow curls. Big curls, like my Boothie has. And he was standing "naked in his own urine." Crying a great big boy. Most nearly a man." She brought her hand up to stop a tear, "And that boy there, he was somebody's son."

> Someone Else's Kids, page 42, Tory Hayden, G.P.
> Putnam's Sons, New York, 1981

Now do you believe me? This is a true story. This really happens. I can tell you what happened to this boy when her mother's brother was in this place too.

He was standing there "naked in his own urine", right?

Do you really think the boy in there just walked in there naked when he was admitted to the place and just went around naked all the time just because he felt like it and urinated all over the place?

No.

I can tell you what happened. The boy went in there fully dressed when he went in there.

What happened was, the staff that worked there "forcibly stripped" this boy of all his clothes including his underwear and stood him in a cell completely naked to the nude. After he was left in there a while with no clothes on, he urinated all over the floor.

They did this to him so everyone in the whole outfit that passed by him would be able to see him completely naked with every inch of his body uncovered including his private area to humiliate him in front of everybody to punish him for being different. They wanted people to see him completely naked. That was the whole purpose. You do something they don't like, and like the Romans they thought, "Well show you!" So, as a result, if you did something they didn't like or they just didn't like your personality, you got stripped. And, in this instance, that meant your underwear too.

They do it for the "power". They do this to suppress the behaviors of their clients they don't like, wrong or not, in order to make them feel inferior to them to force them to be what they want, rather than let them be the way they are freely. They treat them like slaves and that's exactly what they are to them. To most staff people of most institutions their patients are nothing but a piece of property they can kick around and make demands toward and the punishment for not doing what they say or being what they want is being stripped of all their clothes in front of everyone to make a mockery out of them and make them feel inferior to them to gain full control over them. This is even true of some medical hospitals.

The male nurses and "serious trended" female nurses are that controlling. They do this to their patients to publicly shame them and feel like all hope is lost and feel like prisoners and slaves.

However, most of this kind of thing usually happens in mental institutions.

You know how I know?

That's what they did to me.

They didn't lock me up. They just stood me in the back of the Cottage living room and demanded I take my clothes off in front of everybody in the room, eleven boys plus any and all male and female staff in the room and put me on display for everyone to look at undressed to punish me for being different.

They did this in order to humiliate me and make me feel inferior to them and feel low beyond end. Only, in my instance at least they let me keep my underwear on.

Most of the time they handed me a short sleeved white undershirt with colored sleeves to wear with my underwear only. But there were times they even made me shed the shirt and stand there in only my underwear.

Brian Evans
90

However, there was one boy in the entire institution they made go down all the way to the nude and he was placed in a sound proof room where they lectured him completely exposed while the boys in the hallway got to look in and saw everything. Two other times four boys were given a towel to wear and that was all. They weren't wearing underwear either.

Outside of that, these two men and a stern woman that did this to their patients where I was at either made their patients wear the shirt tail shirt and underwear only or made them shed the shirt tail shirt and only go in their underwear in front of everybody if they were upset with them. They did this to me and I was their favorite victim.

That was the mental institution I was in that did this to me.

This story is about a totally different institution.

Mine was not an asylum, but just a general mental institution for boys that had problems with things such as getting in fights with other boys, back talking teachers or parents, and throwing fits, and all the general everyday stuff you see with guy bullies or guys that are picked on by other bullies that can't take it and fight back like I did.

Would you like to know why mental health staffs forcibly strip their patients of their clothes?

Their theory is that if a patient displays unwanted bad behavior that if they embarrass them bad enough they will behave themselves.

They also believe if a patient does something they don't like, wrong or not, if they just don't like their personality that if they embarrass them bad enough they'll never want to do whatever it was that annoys them ever again whether what they did was wrong or not.

So, because of this belief they can make their patients what they want to be whether they did anything wrong or not if they embarrass them to death so they forcibly strip their patients of all their clothes to make a mockery out of them in order to make them what they what them to be instead of how they could be.

It's a control thing. These people are control freaks and that's how they control their patients. They use fear and humiliation as a tool to make them what they want to be instead of letting them be themselves.

I think the only reason I don't remember the men at the military hospital actually forcibly stripping me of my clothes is because I was too afraid of them to refuse to undress for them when they demanded I do so for them. Technically, it was their job to make me change into a hospital gown for examinations but the way they went about getting me to do so for them was bad bedside manner. They could have nicely asked me to do what they needed me to do but instead they yelled at me and demanded I do what they said and glared at me while I undressed myself in front of them like I was dirt to them. When nurses treat you with that kind of inhumane behavior that can actually qualify for being "cruel and unusual punishment". The same goes for the "serious trended" female nurses who yelled at me and forcibly stripped me of my clothes before they tortured me with needles like the men did. What they did was totally uncalled for and was completely cruel.

These men did tackle me down themselves and pinned me down a lot when I was a kid. They were very forceful with me, rammed needles in me, griped at me for screaming and insisted I needed to "bite the bullet" and be a man.

They would yell at me, "I can't take any of your squeamishness or squirminess! You're going to have to bite the bullet! Don't be giving me any trouble! Be still! Do you want to be a problem?! Quit screaming! Come back here you! Be still! Do we have a baby in here?! Do we have a baby in here?! Quit being such a baby! Come on you! I need you to cooperate with me! I'm trying to give you a shot! You better be still or I'll make your life miserable! You need to bite the bullet! Come on! What a baby!"

The proof, my mother knows they did this. She saw it with her own eyes. She didn't see everything these women did, but she did see everything these men did and was not very happy about it.

Most of what happened here was during my Elementary and early Junior High School Years.

Now for the third thing, there really were two men and a stern woman that worked at the institution in authority over me that demanded I take my clothes off in front of a room full of boys.

All of them got to watch me take my shirt and pants and shoes and socks off right in front of them and then one of these three individuals would hand me a white undershirt with colored short sleeves and then said, "Put this on!" These three individuals took turns doing this to me continually to get back at me for being different.

To help you picture what was going on here, if I did something to make you mad at your office and you made me take my clothes off in front of every patient in your lobby to punish me for it that would be terrible, right? That's what these people were doing.

And, it was two men and a stern woman that did this to me and a chipper female staff that protected me from one of the men for the temporary period of time she was there after I already lived there for 10 months. She was only there 2 ½ months and then she was gone. Then, they all had free reign over me again.

Brian Evans
93

See if that makes you see what they were doing. They did this to me in front of eleven boys and every male and/or female staff in the room.

The man with blonde hair, the man with black hair, and the woman with dark red hair that did this to me were not prepping me for a procedure or an examination. They were doing this to make a mockery out of me in front of a room full of boys by putting me on display for them to look at undressed.

They wanted to humiliate the tar out of me and did a good job of it.

The blonde, heavy set male staff and the dark complected, slim railed male staff with black hair also accused me of lying about things all the time.

These two men would take me in their office to lecture me. If I tried to argue with them they would yell, "Brian! Take your clothes off!" They expected me to obey them on the spot.

They would make condescending comments toward me and make a show out of getting to see me naked in front of them.

They would say things to each other like "Let's see what he thinks of himself now! I don't think he'll be giving us any more problems! He's afraid of us now! I don't think he feels too hot about himself without his clothes on! Let's see how we feels now!"

The blonde, heavy set male staff even told me to take my clothes off in front of a female nurse after I hugged her several times in a field outside the cottage. He did this to get back at me for being different.

This lady watched as I took my shirt and my pants and shoes and socks off in front of her and him. She got to stare at me in only me underwear and grinned about it like it gave her pleasure to get back at me.

Brian Evans

Then this man handed me a shirt tail shirt and demanded I put it on over my chest. He lectured me in his office in front of her while I stood there in only my underwear.

After this blonde haired man got me in a shirt tail shirt and my underwear only he bragged about it to this lady and said, "Well Carol! Look what we have here!" in a sarcastic tone of voice and made fun of me.

One time, the slim dark complected male staff with black hair told me to take my clothes off in front of a room full of boys.

He bragged about it and said, "Let's see what you think of yourself now! I bet you don't feel so hot about yourself without your clothes on!"

Later, this male staff with the black hair that had to spoon feed me a lot at meals said, "If you don't start eating right, we're going to make you get an IV! I don't think you'd like that much! So, if you don't want an IV you better start eating right or that's what you are going to get!"

The blonde guy and the black haired guy both spoon fed me but the black haired one is the one that made this sarcastic, threatening comment.

The stern acting slim lady with short, dark red hair that worked there got mad at me for wearing socks to bed one day.

This lady dragged me out of my bedroom into the lobby next to the closet behind the couch and yelled, "Take your clothes off! Now! You broke the curfew, so you can just sit there in front of the closet door in your underwear Indian style now!"

I did this because I was shy about my feet.

That time she didn't even let me wear the shirt tail shirt. She demanded I sit in front of a closet door facing the living room in my underwear only.

One time she made me take my clothes off in front of everybody for asking to get out of playing the games outside.

All of them got to watch while I took my shirt and pants and shoes and socks off right in front of them. This lady did the same thing to me as the men. She didn't do this different just because she was a woman. She did it too, and she was the one that demanded I do this. She got to watch as well as everyone else. Don't think she didn't watch or see anything just because she was a woman.

She did this too and she did it in exactly the same manner as the men did this to me. Nothing was different about the way this was done. That time she let me wear the shirt tail shirt. I still only had my underwear on with the shirt tail shirt she made me wear.

One time I complained to another patient about her on the sidewalk. I got mad and said, "Sherry is a thing of rags!" This lady dragged me in the door and across the room and yelled, "What did you call me?! Is there something you want to say about me?! Take your clothes off now!"

I called her that because she acted like a witch all the time.

That time she also made me go in a shirt tail shirt and my underwear only. As before, she made me do this in front of her and everybody else while she watched. I wasn't exempt from having to do this for her. She did this to me too and she didn't care either.

She made it obvious she hated my guts and she loved it when she made me do this in front of her and everybody else. It made her feel powerful.

This red headed lady constantly had soap box meetings to cut the other patients down.

Brian Evans
96

At four of these soap box meetings she selected certain other patients to also force the shirt tail punishment on.

At two of these meetings she made me take my clothes off in front of everybody and did not give me the shirt tail shirt. She only let me wear my underwear in front of everybody. So I had to go bare-chested and barelegged and barefooted in front of everybody that time and only got to wear my underwear.

The other two times this redheaded lady made me wear a shirt tail shirt and my underwear only. At least I got to wear a shirt tail shirt with my underwear those two times so my chest was covered.

And, this redheaded lady was a stern, cranky woman. She came into the room to call one of her soap box meetings where she sat on a cedar chest. She made us sit around the living room on the couch and in the floor while she lectured us.

When she got everyone seated she yelled, "Don't mess with me or I will make your life miserable! I'm an ex-army cadet and I can be tough so don't mess with me! You better do what I say or else! So don't anybody start on me because I'm not going to take any flack from anybody!" This is a "serious trended" female staff, of course. This lady was also worse than the "Wicked Witch of the West".

That was her way of threatening you that she was going to make you take your clothes of in front of everybody including her if you crossed the line with her and did something she didn't like.
Go figure, huh?

Trust me. She sure wasn't chipper and she never smiled.

The proof: My mother knows they did it and has known it for 3 1/3rd decades.

All you would have to do is call my mother and ask her "Did these two men and this one woman really do this to him at the institute?" and she would tell you I'm telling the truth.

Brian Evans

Not only does she know I'm telling the truth, but one day she saw the red headed staff lady she couldn't stand either and said, "I want to see my son!"

The red headed lady told my mother, "Don't go back there! You might see someone naked!"

My mother said, "I don't care! I'm going back there to see him anyway! I want to see my son!"

My mother said she saw two boys back there with barely anything on and she thought they must have been in their night clothes.

After she told me this, I thought, "I wonder why? Did that horrible red headed woman make these boys take their clothes off and put on a shirt tail shirt in front of everybody before she got there?

I wasn't the only one she ever did this to. I was just the main one they did this to. This lady was very hateful and nobody liked this lady. None of the boys liked her. She was that mean.

If you asked my mother, "Did they in fact make this guy take his clothes off in front of a room full of boys every time he did the least little thing they didn't like?" her answer would be, "Yes! They did!"

Now for the fourth point, notice I said I was afraid this heavy set blonde man would make me take my clothes off in front of everybody if this nice chipper acting lady with long brown hair that came along 10 months after I went in the institution was "not there".

Notice I said, "He refrained from making me take my clothes off in front of her because he was afraid she would get him in trouble for it".

You're probably thinking, "That's because she was a woman."

Really, she was the only woman he wouldn't do this in front of. He made me take my clothes off in front of a female nurse to punish me in front of her.

He didn't care if he made me take my clothes off in front of the stern red headed female staff I told you about either.

But, he did care if he did it in front of this chipper acting lady that liked me.

That's because he feared she would get him in trouble if she caught him doing this because she didn't approve of what he was doing.

This lady had light brown hair, and was slim but slightly broad in the shoulders. I think she said she was 23 years old.

Remember, I was only 14 and she was almost twice my height.

Here's a fifth point. To me a foot massage is a foot massage. When I rubbed this lady's feet it just felt soft on my hands and it relaxed me and that was it.

Here's the question for the people out there who tend to be judgmental: If you really think my rubbing this lady's feet was sexual, then why was I celebrating that I got to keep my clothes on when she was there because she was preventing another man from making me undress myself in front of a room full of boys?

This lady protected me from this heavy set blonde man. Had she not been there, this man would have made me take all my clothes off except my underwear right in front of everybody.

If there was anything sexual going on she would have egged him on, but she didn't. She protected me from this man.

This 30 year old, heavy set, man with wavy blonde hair didn't care if there was another lady hanging around or not either.

This blonde haired man just cared if this particular lady was there because he knew she did not approve and would get him in trouble for doing this to me.

I don't even know where people get the idea this is sexual to begin with. Rubbing someone's feet does not make me feel sexual at all. And, I never heard of it making anyone else feel sexual either.

I can't believe some of these people you run into these days that think everything means something sexual. I never heard anything so ridiculous in my whole life.

They need to get their head out of the gutter.

This never affected me this way. Even most people out there that already know I have a foot fetish think this kind of thing is ridiculous. They never would have seen it that way either.

It's just some of these strange people out there that think this way, not me, and not my friends either. To me, a foot massage is a foot massage.

You can go to the beauty shop to get the same thing done from a pedicurist and no one ever thinks another thing of it because nobody is thinking anything like that.

They know nothing is going on so nobody's worried about it.

If they're not worried about that there, they shouldn't be worried about it here. I was 14 years old when I did this and this was my care taker.

This isn't any worse than a little boy giving a shoe shine to an older man.

To me, giving a lady a foot massage like this would just be another act of kindness that would be greatly appreciated on their part and not thought of in some horrible way.

Brian Evans

Come to think of it, don't you nurses do this for some of your patients anyway?

If you're not worried about this when you do this for your patients, the ones of you that do, it shouldn't be worrisome that I did this for this lady when I was a kid.

To me petting this lady's feet felt like petting a cat. All it did for me is feel soft on my hands and make me relax.

If I had my way all my lady friends would go barefoot and let me give them foot massages. Most of them go barefoot anyway.

I wouldn't mean any harm by it. The reason I would be doing this is to calm my nerves, make my hands feel softer, and relax myself and make them feel happy.

A lot of ladies ask for foot rubs when they need one.

I don't see what the big deal is anyway.

This lady at the institution was a "chipper acting, cheery female" staff person who stood up for me.

She protected me from the man who really did want to do something wrong.

Here's a sixth point. I liked this lady's feet and ever since this lady left I wanted to see every lady's feet and toes and loved it when I got to see them. Before this lady left I never felt this way about it. For one thing, lady's feet are like flowers to me and their toes are like the petals.

Here's my seventh point. This lady was my "protection" against this heavy set blonde man. My parents did not live there, I did. This lady was the only person I could turn to for help.

She was my protection and she was my friend.

Brian Evans

She was the only staff member in the whole institution that liked to go barefoot and let her patients rub her feet.

If you remember another guy patient got me started on it while this lady was there it was still April. School was still going.

What struck me strange all these years is why did this not become an obsession to me immediately?

Why is it that I didn't feel like I had to see my girlfriend's feet at school, especially in desperation to see?

Why not anyone else at school? However, none of them went barefoot anyway.

Then, look at this. I saw my girlfriend at the Rose Park Swimming Pool that summer in June. I saw her feet and her toes and I liked what they looked like. I still wasn't just dying to see them a second time.

It wasn't like it was a desperate thing for me to see them even though I liked them.

Notice, this lady is still at the institution for a couple more weeks.

Then, this lady who was the "protection" against the heavy set blonde man at the institute suddenly leaves.

She quits her job because she doesn't like the way the staff treat their patients.

The heavy set blonde man; the slim, dark complected man with black hair; and, the slim, red headed, stern acting woman who bragged bout being an ex-army cadet now had free reign over me again. They could do whatever they wished to do to me again. This lady who protected me from the blonde man of the bunch was not there to stop him. This nicer lady who protected me while she was there had taken the stern lady's place while she was gone.

Brian Evans
102

Now the stern lady was back. And, now the heavy set blonde man did not have this nice lady around to stop him from punishing me so he was no longer afraid to humiliate me in front of a room full of boys again.

Now that the protection was gone, he did so delightfully just as he did before. So did his dark complected, buddy with black hair. And, so did the redheaded stern lady that worked there.

They all humiliated me in front of everybody in the cottage on a continual basis by demanding I take my clothes off in front of them so everyone in the room would see me in my underwear, just like they did to me before this lady that left had come on the scene.

For the first time ever in July, this blonde man and this black haired man actually took me to my church I attended before I went into the institution. Now I'm out where there are other girls I know that I like and for the first time ever this is when I feel like I've desperately got to see their feet and their toes or I'm going to bust. It was very rare for these guys to take anyone to church too. I think what happened is, was, this lady was my "protection" against the heavy set blonde man.

This lady has now left the institution. The "protection" is now gone.

Now, these girls I was desperate to see the feet became my "protection" against the heavy set blonde man because I did not leave the institution till the following October.

That July, I actually walked up stairs in a gym to see a movie my church was showing. I urgently tried to see the feet and the toes of the first girl I saw wearing sandals. Then, I skipped up the stairs to the next girl gazing down at her feet and toes. Then, I skipped the rest of the way up the stairs, in the entry, and around the corner desperate to see which other girls were showing their feet and their toes.

I was overjoyed when I found to my amazement that several of the girls seated to watch the movie were wearing open toe sandals and I got to see all their feet and toes and felt relieved.

This had never happened to me ever before. As a matter of fact, I didn't even go in there hoping to see girls in their bare feet when I first walked in the door.

It wasn't until I spotted the very first girl in her bare feet on the stair case that I got excited and felt like I had to dash up the stairs from one girl to the next to see who was barefooted and who wasn't. Something went haywire in my brain and all of a sudden it was urgent I got to see every girls' bare feet and toes that I could and I couldn't even figure out why it was urgent I got to see them. I think it must have freaked me out that Jenny left the institution four months before I got out and now I was stuck with having to deal with the heavy set blonde male staff continually making me take my clothes off in front of a room full of boys to humiliate me again. When this happened I had to skip up the stairs from one girl to the other to see them in sandals because for the first time ever it was suddenly urgent I had to see. It was just an automatic reaction I had to being able to see a girl in their bare feet that I never had before. This never mattered to me before this. But for some reason, on this day, it was urgent I got to see every girl's feet and toes. When I did, I was incredibly relieved. I felt like I was about to rejoice and celebrate. It was like consciously I was thinking, "Alright! Feet!" but subconsciously I was thinking "They'll protect me! That heavy set blonde man won't get me when their around!" That's the way I felt. My emotions had now gone from "Scat your feet!" to "Please! I've got to see your toes! It's driving me crazy!"

So, from that day forward, I was desperate to see every lady's and girl's feet and toes or I was going to bust and this has been a problem since.

Girls always had to protect me from the boys and the men during my Elementary and Junior High School years.

I was constantly being bullied by someone and they always had to step in to protect me or I'd get jumped by another boy or harassed by a male adult.

My female peers and female teachers constantly had to protect me in school from other boys and male teachers all throughout my Elementary and Junior High School years. I was also short for my age. I was only 14 years old and I was only 5'1" on the day this happened. When I went into the institution at 13 I was only 4'7". I didn't even reach 5'3" till several months later when I turned 15 in March of the following year.

I think I was "traumatically shocked" into being this way.

Before I met this lady, I demanded that every girl or lady I saw barefoot put their shoes back on and cover their feet. "Now I feel like I have to beg every girl and lady to take their shoes and socks off and let me see their feet and their toes."

Now it's urgent I get to see their toes and I feel like I'm going to go bananas if I don't.

Strange isn't it?

I think this is what caused this to happen.

It's almost like "the barefooted lady saved the day".

So, if you're someone who likes to go barefoot in flip flops or sandals and you see me staring at your feet, please do not be alarmed. I just like to be able to see every lady's feet and toes because they look like pretty flowers to me. I mean nothing amiss by this.

And, if you are someone who likes to go barefoot but wears closed toe shoes, don't be surprised if I look at you nervously, looking down at your feet longingly acting like something is wrong.

Brian Evans
105

When I do this it is because I like ladies' feet and I want to be able to see your toes and you are hiding your toes causing me not to be able to see what looks like the petals of the flowers. I'm like a kid in a candy store that thinks, "I want to see! I want to see!"

So, please don't see me as an adult male acting like this but as a child in a man's body acting like this.

I'm kind of the same way with this as Rain Man is with his camera.

I really can't help it that I'm like this because I am autistic, so please don't use it against me. It's just the way I am. I've been like this since I was 14 years old. However, I've been autistic since I was born.

And if I ever ask to see your toes please do not scold me for this because in reality it is a child inside of a man's body that is thinking this and acting this way. It actually makes me sad to not be able to see your feet and your toes.

It's actually kind of unfair in a way, if you asked me to show you my feet you would expect me to obey you but if I ever asked to see yours I might be in trouble, but I might not, it depends on how you react.

If it does bother you that I've asked to see your feet and your toes please do not refrain from examining my feet when I have problems with them, because I still need you to tend to them when things go wrong. Right now, the main problem I keep having is ingrown toenails, bending toe nails, and breaking toe nails. So, if something of this nature happens and it gets really bad I really need you to look at it to see what you can do to treat them if they're really messed up that day.

Please do not let my wanting to see your feet and toes stop you from examining mine when a foot examination is necessary for me to have when I have problems with my feet or toenails. I promise I mean no harm. I'm just trying to get you to treat me for whatever is wrong with my feet when this happens. I'm sorry if this makes you uncomfortable. Thank you.

This is what I was referring to in "To Nurse Means to Nurture Part 2" that I thought some nurses would think was cute that other nurses would think was horrible if I brought it up to them.

I feared the nurses that didn't understand all this would scold me to death, but figured that other nurses would know I was just being silly and say, "Oh, that's just him, leave him be." Believe it or not, it's nothing personal. I'd be the same way if you were a stranger in a grocery store. I'm this way with everybody. This is not unusual and you have nothing to worry about because I'm not singling you out because you are nurses. This is what I was referring to that was not on my list of needs that I have a hang-up with that some nurses would think was cute and others would think was horrible.

I figured you would think, "What does this have to do with us?" but I just wanted you to know what was going on when I am like this and help you understand why I am this way. This section explains all this to help you understand. I hope you understand. Please do not be angry about this section. I just wanted you to see for a few pages how this particular hang-up with my autism affects me before I go on about the Emergency Room and ICU section of the book. The moral of the story is, don't let my hang-ups make you not meet my list of needs. I don't want you to stop meeting my list of needs just because you are aggravated with me about my hang-ups. Like, I said, this particular hang-up I have I thought you would hate the worst about me is not even that personal, it just looks that way. Like I said, I'd be the same way if you were a stranger in a grocery store.

Brian Evans
107

It's not because you are a nurse I'm asking you this if I ever do, it's because I'm that way with everybody and you just happen to be one of the everybody's out there there is I'm this way with in addition to everybody else. That is everybody else that's a lady everywhere else. I'm only that way with ladies, not men. I really don't even like men. I have a few laid back guy friends but almost all of my friends are ladies.

Please keep reading and try to understand. I'm autistic and mean no harm at all by this. Thank you.

After all these years that all these nurses made me go barefooted in front of them whether I liked it or not, toes and all, I ought to be able to see yours.

I actually saw several nurses wearing flip flops at a place I went a few years ago I had to get a test at and even the ones that came for me were wearing flip flops and I got to see their feet and their toes and I liked it.

That was the first time ever I ever saw any nurse wear flip flops or even go barefooted at all. Before that they all wore shoes and socks, but I didn't care because I thought their feet looked pretty.

I guess you figured out by now that a lady's toes are my favorite part. Getting to see the feet without the toes is like looking at the stem to a flower without getting to see the petals.

Can you see how disappointing that would be not to be able to see somebody's toes if that's the way you felt about it?

I even saw a few receptionists at the hospital I went to for 10 years that was so nice to me until they got new nurses that were wearing sandals and flip flops and I was amazed. I thought, "Wow! This is different! They're even wearing sandals and going barefoot."

Not long after that I even saw one of my younger PreOp nurses at that hospital walking down the Radiology hall in sandals to the PreOp department. I thought, "Wow! This is different! I never thought one of my PreOp nurses would wear sandals to the hospital!"

Then, to my amazement, a few days later, when Bertha had to go set up a mammogram at that hospital in 2015 one of my Radiologist's I was friends with was working as a receptionist for the Mammography office and she was wearing open toe sandals too. I believe hers were flip flops too.

I thought, "Wow! This gets better every minute! I thought I'd never see the day when my own nurses went around barefooted! They always made me go barefooted in front of them every time I turned around whether I liked it or not toes and all when I was younger and now I'm getting to see them go barefooted for once. It's like the tables turned now. After all these years of nurses making me go barefooted in front of them toes and all and acting gruff about it it's like a relief to be able to see nurses being the ones that go barefooted. The only difference is, they do this because they feel like it. I did it because I had to.

This hospital I went to for 10 years nearly always let me wear my socks because they knew I was shy about my feet, but the last time I went to their GI department they wouldn't let me wear my socks in there anymore and got to see me in my bare feet toes and all just like the military hospital and the institution did. They didn't even give me those hospital socks you get in a Pre-Op setting sometimes. Only I've noticed some places give you those and some don't.

The last time I went to their PreOp department for my last procedure there they almost didn't let me wear my socks then. They really wanted me to go barefooted but Bertha talked them into letting me wear my socks. I think they changed the rules and said "No socks aloud." like hospitals used to do.

Brian Evans
109

Some places let you wear your socks and other places make you take them off whether you like it or not and they don't care how you feel about it, they just expect you to do it.

Nurses are actually more pleasant to be around when they wear flip flops but they still have to be chipper acting ones or this don't count. I don't feel as much like a Guiney pig when they go barefooted in flip flops and open toe sandals.

I feel like they are more on my level and less scary to be around when they wear sandals and show their toes.

It's like they're one big happy family and their laid back and it feels like they might as well say, "Hey, we have feet and toes too. Don't feel bad that you have to go barefooted in front of us part of the time or wear hospital gowns with no socks. We like to go barefoot too. So, don't be ashamed."
It was even scarier to be around nurses when they wore those white smocks, white hats, and white tennis shoes. When they quit wearing those scary outfits and got more casual and started wearing those multicolored design tops and tennis shoes that was much less scary and it felt more like being around nurse mommies that are there to take care of you and help you through the scary stuff to make it not so bad. And, when some of them started getting even more casual and wearing sandals and showed their toes it started feeling like, "Hey. We're laid back here. Just relax. We're your friends and we're going to take care of you." It also felt like, "Don't be ashamed you have to go barefoot or wear gowns in front of us sometimes. We're barefoot too. See. There's nothing to be ashamed of."

It helps when they are wearing sandals and you don't feel like the naked peon slave in front of them when they're dressed up all fancy and you're not. Even if I get to keep my clothes on or don't have to take my shoes and socks off in front of them it still helps me feel more at ease with them when they wear sandals and show their toes.

Brian Evans

When someone wears slip on shoes it drives me crazy and I feel like begging them to take them off. If they ever do, I feel like, "Thank God, they're barefoot! What a relief!" They are more pleasant to be around when they're the chipper acting cheery females that are wearing flip flops or sandals so you can see their toes.

Most of them wear tennis shoes and that's fine too, but when they do wear sandals it makes me feel very pleased and helps me relax more.

There was one nurse I think caught on that I liked this that actually did wear flip flops in front of me recently that I got the feeling thought, "I know he likes this. Maybe if I do this I won't have to meet his list of needs as much." Sorry, that doesn't count.
I have to have my list of needs met whether you go barefoot in front of me to make me happy or not, if that's what you're doing. That's what I suspected was going on, anyway.

If you do go barefooted, please let me see your toes, but if it's going to offend you please don't let this stop you from being my nurse. Please don't reject me. I don't want to lose you.
And, please don't be angry with me for this if it offends you.

Please don't shy away from me just because you read this or start acting cold toward me or acting formal.

If you do, I won't be sticking around.

I can't handle not being able to have the nurses I like. I want chipper acting, cheery females only and no one else will do.
I cannot take a male or serious trended female nurse.

And, if you're a nurse that never goes barefooted around people to begin with please don't worry about this if you see this. I might like it better if you did go barefooted but I'm not going to make you do anything you don't want to do.

Brian Evans
111

I'm mainly talking to the nurses and receptionists that already go barefooted in shoes without socks; mainly slip on shoes that I wish would wear sandals or flip flops instead.

If my family doctor is reading this, please don't be angry with me. I don't' want to be in trouble with you. I love my family doctor and I don't want to do anything to offend her. She is like a mother figure to me and I don't want to lose her if I offend her.

She is my favorite doctor and she is the most wonderful doctor I ever met in the whole world and I couldn't handle it if I lost her. Please remember the person I quoted out of one of the college textbooks of nursing I found that says, "Regardless of the fact that what you said makes me uncomfortable I still accept you." I want you to accept me no matter what I do and treat me the same as you always have. Please, I beg you not to be angry with me. I can't help it if I slip up every now and then with something like this. I'd still like you to wear sandals if it didn't bother you to do so for me but I don't want to make you mad by asking you if you could so I'm scared to ask. I have a hang up in this area because of my Autism. I don't mean anything bad by it.

Please don't be angry at me for this. Please try to understand me. I don't mean any harm at all. I'm not singling you out like it may look like I am. If I had my way every girl and every lady everywhere I go would wear open toe sandals. It's nothing personal at all. I don't want you to be offended that I want to see your toes. I want you to be honored I want to see your toes. And, the same goes for all other lady's I want to see the toes of. Please try to understand and please forgive me if this offends you.

If any of my other nurses that I currently go to are reading this, please don't be angry with me. I love you guys too.

And, please don't stop going barefooted just because you read this. I'd rather you go ahead and wear your slip on shoes with no socks than to wear boots to work and make me feel like I'm being punished for asking to see your toes.

Brian Evans
112

I like the bright neon colored slip on shoes anyway. I just like to see everyone's toes better. It's not just you. I want to see every lady's toes everywhere I go, no matter where it is. You don't have to be a nurse for me to feel this way. I'm this way with everybody. All my lady friends know this. I just wanted you to know this so you would understand me. My lady friends already understand I am this way and it does not bother them at all. They think it's cute and sweet.

If it makes my family doctor and all of my nurses at my specialist's offices and hospital nurses feel any better I told my Psychology teacher friend Bertha does speeches for that I was this way about lady's feet and both her and her younger students in her office wore open toe sandals just for me because they knew I was that way and wanted to make me happy. It did not bother them at all.
They knew I had no bad intentions for this and were more than happy to do this for me. They thought it was sweet and they thought it was cute. And, I know most of you hospital nurses don't go barefoot and usually wear tennis shoes all the time. That's fine. I'm not telling you to do anything different.

Most of the ones that like to go barefoot work at offices, but if you do work in the hospital and run around barefoot in slip on shoes, please wear sandals instead so I can see your toes if it doesn't bother you to do this for me. Thank you. I'm sorry if this embarrasses you. It's embarrassing for me to talk about or tell you about too.

Please do not hold this against me and see it for what it is and that is just another hang-up due to my Autism I have that causes me to be this way. The best way to relieve my anxiety over not being able to see your toes would be to either take your slip on shoes off or put on flip flops or open toe sandals, unfortunately. I'm sorry.

Brian Evans
113

So, if this really bothers you, don't let it bother you, just blow it off and go on and please treat me with the same tenderly comfort and compassion you always do in the same way you always do for me without condemning me and act like this never whole thing never happened. So, please keep that in mind when you read all this stuff I have here about this. You're not the only ones.

Last summer, Bertha had a ladies' meeting at our house and every one of the ladies were barefooted in flip flops and open toe sandals and I liked it.

They were very pleasant to be around and it made me really happy because that's my favorite way for ladies to be is barefoot. I don't mean anything bad by it. I'm just that way.

Please don't reject me. Please don't shun me away.

I'm autistic and I mean absolutely no harm by this. It's just another hang-up I have that drives me up the wall like having to have the furniture arranged a certain way or have all Christmas colored walls and floors, have Christmas decorations, and trinkets, and dolls all over the house.

Believe it or not, even my peers in high school asked to see the feet and toes of other peers and they had all their factors unlike me.

They would all ask each other, "What do yours look like? What do yours look like?" and compare them and compliment each other about their feet and their toes. They thought it was neat.

One guy said to a girl, "What do yours look like?" and when the girl showed him he said, "Oh, you have crunchy toes."

The first girl was already wearing sandals.

Most of the others they asked were actually wearing their shoes and socks.

Brian Evans
114

They actually took their shoes and socks off to show their peers that asked them to let them see their feet and showed them their feet and toes to make them happy. And, they weren't upset at all.

They were very happy to show them what they looked like. They thought it was cute and neat.

Several others wore sandals already and the other boys and girls would always look at each other's feet and compare their feet and toes with each other and make comments.

Most of them were just being silly, but they didn't mean a thing bad by it. They just thought it was neat and they just wanted to see them out of curiosity.

These were actually boys and girls at a church youth retreat.

Boys and girls both asked another girl student in class to show them her feet because she was talking about her toes and they wanted to know what they looked like.

Believe it or not, the girl took her shoe and sock off just to show them so they could see her toes and said, "See. Here's what they look like. The second one is longer than the first."

The only problem is I get grossed out when the second toe is longer than the first.

This girl did this in front of her whole class at school.

If their toes are perfectly aligned from big to small from the big toe to the pinky in a half circle then I like them. When they look like that and are perfectly shaped, then they look pretty and look like petals on flowers. I love to see every girl's and lady's toes when they look like this.

I don't understand why I have to be punished for wanting to see everybody's feet and toes if my high school peers with all their factors can ask to see each other's feet and toes and not get in trouble with anybody for it or make anybody mad. They did it gladly for each other. Most of them were being silly.

They didn't mean anything by this when they did this and I don't mean anything bad by this either. I just want to see.

Please don't be upset with me for this.

When I ask you, "Can I see your toes?" or "Can you wear sandals the next time?" if you're wearing slip on shoes with no socks please see a child. Why would a child ask you if they could see your toes? Why would a child ask you if you could wear sandals the next time?

The reason they would want you to wear sandals and see your toes is the same reason I would want you to wear sandals and see you toes.

I'm actually a sweet little boy that's asking you this that's trying to come out because he's a child in a man's body. Please try to see this. I mean no harm.

Because of my disability I don't think like other men.

Even Bertha said once, "You're funny! Forget what other men like to look at; you just want to see their feet. You're sure not like them, but I like you better that way. I'd rather you want to look at somebody's feet than something else. I never saw anything like it. You're a mess."

I actually look at Collections, Etc., ABC Distributing and LTD Commodities Catalogues just to see lady's feet.

I've just got to see lady's feet and their toes and all of these are Christmas catalogues with Christmas trinkets and decorations and dolls and women's Caftan's, pajamas, and dresses show lady's with their feet uncovered and their toes showing. All of them are descent. All of them are barefooted. And, all of them are showing their toes. I look like crazy through these catalogues to see them.

I usually find several of them in the Collections Etc. Catalogues and I usually stare intently at all of them because I think their pretty.

I even wait around for Vana White commercials on Wheel of Fortune to run to the TV to see her feet and toes because she wears slip on shoes during the show but she usually wears flip flops during nearly all her commercials.

I even watch kid movies looking for movies with girls that go barefoot in them so I can see their feet and toes too.

Don't worry; I don't just watch these movies for the feet only. I have always liked kid movies that are nearly always about girls whether their barefooted or not, but if they are barefooted I like it all the better.

I even looked at an AVON catalogue last Christmas gazing at this picture of a ladies bare foot that showed their toes and there wasn't even a person connected to it in the picture. They just showed the foot and I still had to desperately see what it looked like.

I want to see every girl's and lady's bare feet and toes so bad that it makes me want to cry when I don't get to see them or they cover up their toes with those slip on shoes. Like I said, I like the slip on shoes, and many of them are pretty, especially the peach ones I saw my favorite doctor wearing but I like to see their toes better. It's not because I'm trying to be over personal with anybody. I just want to see their toes because it drives me crazy not to see them because I love every girl's and lady's toes. So please do not be offended by this. It is just my autism.

Brian Evans
117

My friends already know I'm this way. If I had my way every girl and lady everywhere would pull their shoes and socks off and wear a pair of flip flops or open toe sandals and 90% of the ones I know I wish this about already do 90% of the time anyway, so it's not like I have to worry about any of them not going barefooted in sandals. They already do.

I just wanted my nurses to know this too so they would know what was going on.

If any of you ever did decide to let me see your feet and your toes I would thank you all over the place.

I'd like to show you how Autism plays into this in the next two quotes and then I'm going to go on to another topic shortly.

"Management guidelines and specialist pre-admission procedures (including an Autistic Anesthetic Questionnaire) are used to elicit specific responses regarding the nature and severity of the child's autism condition (such as severity; developmental level; likes/fetishes/dislikes; phobias for food, drink, activities and objects; special needs; medication, general health; and social/home circumstances). The admission process is individualized to meet the specific needs of the patient."
>   Health Care and the Autism Spectrum: A Guide For Health
>   Professionals, Parents and Carers, Alison Morton-Cooper,
>   Jessica Kingsley Publishers, 2004

I believe all this is a result of my autism.

"Autism – (definition "e") – bizarre experiences to various aspects of the environment (e.g., resistance to change; "peculiar interest in or attachments to inanimate objects."
>   Terminology of Communication Disorders, Speech-
>   Language Hearing, Nicolosi, Harryman, Kresheck,
>   Williams & Wilkins, A Waverly Company, 1989, page 33

Here is an example of an autistic person being obsessed with inanimate objects:

"Then there is the fascination with bright lights, or with strange objects such as bits of broken plastic or elastic bands."
 Funk & Wagnall's New Encyclopedia of Illustrated Family Health, Marshall Cavendish Limited, 1988, page 108

You see, in this instance my peculiar interest in an inanimate object would be my fascination with lady's feet, mainly their toes.

And the same goes for Christmas trees, bright colors, Christmas colored walls and floors, Christmas Decorations, Antique Dolls, Kid movies, Board games, Tea Parties, Quilts, and the like.

If you notice all of my interests in these areas are all like that of a kid or a girl.
I'm not much like a guy at all and when I was a kid the other guys always called me a sissy.

I also got jumped a lot by boys and treated with cruelty by male doctors, male nurses, male teachers, and many other male authority figures.

I hope this explains some of my weirdness I fear you think I have.

Please do not be upset about anything I said here.

And please do not let any of this knowledge of what I've told you here keep you from being my nurse.

I will take "chipper acting cheery female nurses" only for my nurses and no one else.

I will never take a "male nurse" or "serious trended female nurse" even if I lose a "chipper acting female nurse" over something like this.

Brian Evans
119

I will walk away the minute any one ever does this to me and you will never see me again, probably not any of you because I will not be coming back if you do this to me.

I want you, my "chipper acting female nurses" to accept me even if something like this bothers you.

Please treat me the same way you always do and continue to meet my list of needs the same way you always do. I want "chipper acting cheery female nurses" only or there's no deal.

I hope you understand.

If any of this same information is brought to your attention by someone else I still want you to accept me the way I am even if they are someone that wants to make a ruckus about something.

Please don't ever let anything anyone says change the way you feel about me.

It just makes me want to cry when I feel like your going to misunderstand me over something like this and I feel like if no one's going to understand I might as well get out of everyone's way.

How can anyone possibly understand something like this?

I wish they could. But, if your going to be cross with me and act all formal and not meet my needs for comfort in the same way you always do or you refuse to be my nurse altogether, I'll just get out of everyone's way and never go to a doctor or hospital ever again. It's too hard for me to bear the rejection I receive from anybody anymore.

Just please don't reject me and stay the same and always be there for me no matter how much I offend you.

Brian Evans
120

I beg you, please don't hold any of this against me, and please don't let my fascination I have with lady's feet due to my Autism keep you from being my nurse. I don't want to lose you.

Please, just accept me the way I am and treat me the way you always have.

I'm sorry if anything I've said here has offended you. I don't want you to be mad I want to see your toes, I want you to be honored I want to see your toes because I think they are pretty like flowers.

So, if this bothers you, just please try to overlook this and remind yourself, "He's just being a kid. He doesn't mean anything by it. He's just acting like a 5 year old again and I just need to deal with it and go on as if he never said anything." Please do this for me. Thanks. Anyway, please keep reading. I want you to hear the rest.

Because this is a book about anxiety, I wanted to let you see how this hang-up I have affects me emotionally so you can understand how important it is to me to see a lady's feet and toes and how much it hurts my feelings to not be able to see them. I was originally just going to briefly let you know I was like this so you would know what to expect but the reason I went ahead and drew this topic out is because I wanted you to be able to see the emotions I have and how much it torments me to feel this way due to my Autism. Whether you consider it appropriate or not, it's still a form of anxiety caused by my Autism. If this person in this book I quoted that wrote a book about Autism and Nursing is telling parents to tell doctors and nurses in the hospital setting what their child's interests and fetishes are, then I ought to be able to tell you what my fetishes are without having to feel like I have to be punished for it.

Please remember this when you take in account what I told you about it and show mercy to me and let me be able to speak my peace about this issue in peace.

Brian Evans

I mean no harm to anybody and this is just a hang-up I have due to my Autism I struggle with and I just wanted to be able to explain it to you.

Like I said, before I met that lady at that institution I rubbed the feet of that protected me from that man that was trying to punish me unjustly by putting me on display undressed in front of a room full of boys for being "goofy" as he claimed I was completely the opposite.

But for some reason, after she left and I was still there for four more months, it's like it threw me into some kind of shock to cause me to be the opposite of the way I originally was.

I literally went from hating feet to loving feet. And, I literally went from demanding people cover their feet to begging them to uncover their feet and let me see their toes after she left. I didn't beg them verbally, but in my mind I did.
This very thing is just now coming out verbally expressed that I felt since Age 14 which was silently unknown to others, but obvious in the way I acted. The only reason I didn't let out the bag about feeling this way until now is because I was too shy to ask someone if they would do this for me or tell them this kind of thing was bothering me. It is an embarrassing subject for me to talk to people about and it makes me feel uncomfortable to discuss it with people because of how embarrassed I am to talk to people about my feet or their feet. I even go to a chiropractor that pulls on my feet and my toes. Each time I'll ask them to pull my toes because my feet and toes tend to get stiff but I actually have to struggle to tell them this is what I want because I am so embarrassed to say the words, "Can you pull my toes?" to them because I feel so ashamed of myself that I have feet and I'm embarrassed to talk to them about mine or theirs even though, I am just dying to see their toes because it drives me crazy not to be able to see them.
 I wish they'd wear sandals too but I'm scared to ask.

I've been this way since Age 14, but I'm just now speaking up about it and struggling to say it, not because I'm guilty of anything but because it embarrasses me to talk about feet to anybody because I am so shy.

So, please, see this for what it is as a state of shock causing an Autistic individual that's like a child in a man's body to be this way.

This was because of a traumatic experience where a nice lady I rubbed the feet of at an institution I was in that protected me from a man trying to continually humiliate me in front of everybody left well before I was discharged.

It was after the day she left that this tendency began in me unknowns to me until the first time I was able to get away where other girls were at that were barefoot that I also thought would protect me from this man.

I was never this way before this lady left. Not during the time she was there did I have this problem except for wanting to pet her feet and not one time before I met her was I ever like this before.

As I said, I was the direct opposite of this before this woman came along. Before I met this lady I demanded all girls cover their feet when I saw them barefoot.

After this boy talked me into petting this lady's feet and she protected me for 2 ½ months from that man at the institution, suddenly I felt like I was begging in my mind for every girl to uncover their feet because I was desperate to see their toes and it was urgent I got to see. I was 14 years old when this happened and I've been this way ever since.

You think all this is bad. At least I don't go to the bowling alley smelling everybody's shoes.

Brian Evans
123

I read something about an autistic individual that went around smelling other people's shoes that were lying around at the bowling alley.

So, before you think evil of me and think, "If another man asked to see my feet and toes they might have evil intentions." remember this, if I had never met this woman who protected me from this man I would never have been like this. Be glad I'm desperate to see your feet and toes and am honored to see them.

If it had not been for her, I would still be demanding every woman cover their feet, but because of this woman I feel like I have to see them uncovered or I'm going to bust. It wasn't for sexual reasons then and it's not for sexual reasons now.

Besides that, I was a kid when this happened and I had barely been 14 for 3 months when she disappeared after my ex-girlfriend also disappeared a week or two before. Now that's a double shock. You see why I'm like this.

So, don't blame me for evil thoughts because some other man out there might think this way because that is not the way I think and that is never the way I thought. Whatever I thought unconsciously since the Age of 14 is the same thing I think now, whatever that may be and it hasn't changed since. It's a "shock"!

You know how some people suddenly can't speak when someone their close to dies.

That's what happened with this when that lady left the institution that protected me from a man that wanted to punish me unjustly using humiliation as a tool.

When she left, that's when the pattern started.

I didn't even know I was going to feel the way I did until the minute the problem first struck me in the very first situation I felt this way in that I didn't even know I was going to feel this way in and normally would not have felt this way in. It didn't bother me before I met this lady, so why did it begin to bother me then when I didn't even expect it? It has to be an act of shock. That's got to be what caused this. I don't know what to say.

I truly believe I was traumatically shocked into being this way. I'm sorry if it offends people. And, I'm sorry if I'm embarrassing any of you. Please forgive me. I know what it's like to be shy about your feet because I am shy about mine.

I'm doing a lot better than I used to where it's okay for some people to see, but that's normally a nurse, and I may be okay with one nurse and completely clam up on another nurse. So, I can see how this can be embarrassing for you, but I have a feeling most of you are not even embarrassed about your feet because you could really care less whether anyone sees your feet or not including your toes. Like most people I know you're probably thinking, "If I decide I want to go barefoot, I'm going to plop my feet right out there, toes and all. I don't care what anybody thinks."

Most people I know feel that way about it, but I do know that some people are shy like I am and I'm sorry if this embarrasses you or offends you. It's not my fault I'm like this and I mean absolutely nothing bad by it. Please have mercy on me and treat me like a child and be willing to see me as a child when I do this because I mean absolutely nothing by it. Thank you.

Remember, this is just a book and I am just trying to educate you on what I am like so you know what to expect so there won't be any unnecessary misunderstandings.

I want you to be able to see me in a different light.

Brian Evans
125

Who is he really? What is he really like? How does he really think? Does he have certain idiosyncrasies and/or sensory issues that we don't have that are hard to make sense of to us?

Does he want various things he asks of us for the same reason a child would ask these things?

Does he really think like an adult when he says or does odd things or is it possible that maybe he's thinking from the mind of a child with childlike thoughts and childlike wants and childlike needs when he says or does things that seem odd to us?

Is it possible that nearly every time he says something to us we need to consider the possibility that he is a child asking us these things with the thoughts of a child, the wants of a child, and the special needs of a child?

Does he need all this attention and affection from us for the same reason a child would?

Is a child in a man's body asking us to do this for him and not a man?

What if we're really not talking to a man at all and we are talking to a child here and he is asking us things from the perspective of a child rather than an adult?

Are we in fact talking to a child every time we talk to this guy?

Does he in fact need us to meet his childlike needs in childlike ways because he really is a child in an adult body? Does he not think like we do and interpret things the way we do?

Does he really see everything through the eyes of a child and all his wishes and wants and desires are the same as a child and every time he desires anything of us that sounds weird to us he is desiring these things from the heart of a child innocently asking things of us we would normally conceive as mischievous when they are totally innocent?

Who is this guy and how does his mind work? Who are we talking to?

Are we really talking to an adult when we take things wrong he says and wish to punish him for worse than death when in fact his motives and intentions are far from mischievous and he is saying things, doing things, and asking things for the same reasons as someone in the stages of infancy? How can this be? Why is he so smart? How can this be if he is so smart?

Is it possible that he is only this smart because he was normalized and memorized a bunch of facts and that is the reason he knows all this stuff about what we are supposed to do for him and how to research it?

So, intellectually from a book perspective he is one of us, but from a social and emotional perspective he is not one of us?

Is he a child in his emotional mind and social thinking and everything that seems odd to us of a mischievous nature is actually innocent because he does not think like us?
Is he actually affected differently by things than the rest of us?

Are some of the things we desire for reasons that are not right things that he desires for reasons that there is nothing wrong with?

It is possible for this to happen depending on the mindset of the person thinking them.

One person can want something for one reason and another want the same thing for a totally different reason.

Brian Evans

Even in the normal world, one person may want a high paying job for the sole purpose of power and control and prestige.

Another person desiring the same job may want this job simply because it is something they enjoy doing and could care less how much power and control and prestige it can give them.

The first person desiring this job is in the wrong, but the second person desiring the same job is in the right because they wanted the job for the right reasons.

If you think about it, it is the same way with you guys.

One person may want to be a nurse because they just want a job where they can receive a paycheck and that's all they care about and they could care less about the patient or what their needs are.

Another person may also want to be a nurse because they love working with people and they have a heart for the sick and the ill and the disabled and the elderly or even children. They want to be able to do everything they can in their might to help these people and care for them. They want to comfort them the best way they can because they love them. They are willing to touch them and hug them and rub their head to calm them down and hold their hand through a needle stick like they need. And they are willing to do anything else they can to comfort them in addition to this they may not have already done for them because they love them. Which one of these individuals is in the right?

Is it the first or the second?

It's obvious the answer is the second, because the first person didn't care anything for the patient and only wanted to be a nurse for the paycheck.

The second person wanted to be a nurse because they love working with people and love helping patients and they wanted to comfort them and care for them all they could because they meant something to them and they loved them.

You see, if you reverse the first example of how a typical person might think into the way the person in the second example might think in both instances, you might see how I think.

Also, one teenager may ask you, "Can I have some paint?" and you say, "Sure" and then they go vandalize a room somewhere.

Another teenager with a different personality might ask you for paint and say, "Can I have some paint?" and all he wants to do is paint a picture on a canvas.

You can't punish the second teenager for what the first teenager did because the second teenager didn't do anything.

The second teenager's motives for wanting the paint were good and right, but the first teenager's motives for wanting the paint were bad.

So, when you punish me for asking you for things you think to be mischievous in nature because another adult might want the same thing for the wrong reasons this is what I feel like.

This is because what I was asking you was out of the goodness of my own heart in sweet sincerity but the other person had evil thoughts.
When you do this to me you're making me suffer the consequences for what the typical person thinks wrong instead of what I think that's not wrong.

So, I feel like you are punishing me for their evil thoughts for asking my odd requests of you because you assume since most other adults mean something bad by the same thing I must mean that too.

Brian Evans
129

Now I'm in trouble because you think I've crossed the line with you when I never meant anything bad by anything I said or did.

You can't punish me for what someone else does or did when I ask you for the same things because I ask you the same question out of innocence that they asked you out of mischievousness.

It's not my fault the other adult wanted the same thing for the wrong reasons. What they did is their own fault, but when you blame me according to what they think when I ask for the same things, I feel like I am being punished for what they did instead of what I truly wanted.

When the light hits and you see who I really am and how I really think and are able to see all my wants and wishes and desires and needs are the same as a child's wants and wishes and desires and needs because I am a child in a man's body asking for these things, wishing for these things, desiring all these things, and needing the childlike things I need because they are genuine needs that are dire needs that need met for the same reason an infant or very young child would need them then you will say to yourself, "We need to take care of this guy as if he were a child and respond to his requests as if he was a child asking us all these things. We need to consider that his desires are the desires of a child, that his wishes are the wishes of a child, and that the needs he has are dire needs that are the genuine needs of a child that have to be met. We need to do this to help him sustain his equilibrium and we need to meet his special needs for hugs and comfort as if he was a child receiving this from us as if we were his mothers."
Besides that, nurses are the "mother surrogates" of the patients they take care of. Those patients, even if they are adults need to be allowed to regress to the level of a child in childlike ways and have their childlike needs met.

And, someone like me, who is already regressed in this way, needs to be able to have these needs met at all times by his nurses no matter what situation he is in.

This is especially true when I am in stressful situations involving pain and fear.

In these cases they need to be willing to meet these needs all the more and flood me with love and affection and comfort to help me through the procedures and inpatient stays in the hospital I have.

This is what I am trying to get you to see.

And, you also need to understand that even the things that are non medical in nature that may not be on my list of needs that sound strange to you are just idiosyncrasies or hang-ups I have and they are also coming from the mind of a child and the reasons behind them are the same as a child's reasons for the same things.

To find out how to best deal with the special needs and odd requests of patients with autism you can ask yourself the following questions: "What are their sensory issues? What are their special needs? What odd things may they say, do, or ask that we might normally take in the wrong context do we need to know about? Do we need to blow these things over and in some instances possibly even play along since they don't mean anything bad by anything they say or do? What should we do to help these people and how should we react to them? What do we need to do to meet their comfort needs? What do we need to take seriously and what do we need to overlook? Maybe we should think about these things when an autistic patient comes our way so we know the best way to keep them happy and the best way to meet all their needs to the best of our ability with all the comfort and reassurance we can give them. Be willing to give them a little slack. These people are different. They don't think like you and me. Let's just accept them for the way they are. We need to overlook all their odd differences with their idiosyncrasies and quirks and accept them the way they are with full love and compassion. They can't help the way they are because they are autistic. That's just the way they are. We just need to adjust to meeting their needs and understanding their personality and accepting them for who they are. This is what we need to do and this is what they need."

Brian Evans
131

My mother wanted me to be taken care of after she dies and in order for this to happen; all my doctors, nurses, and techs in the hospital setting and doctor's offices need to be willing to give me hugs. I have to receive chipper acting female nurses and techs only. No males and no serious trended females of any kind.

A chipper acting female nurse has to rub my head to calm me down through needle sticks such as IVs, Blood Tests, Shots, Biopsies, Tube insertions, catheters, or anything else sharp.
I need to be put completely to sleep for all invasive procedures.
This also includes catheters and tube insertions, even urinary catheters and stomach tubes and heart catheters. I cannot be awake for this and have to be numb for this.

Also, I need all my nurses to not only to meet all my emotional needs for comfort but also be willing to accept all my idiosyncrasies and sensory issues I have and accept me the way I am as a disabled individual. They need to be willing to not punish me for things that sound strange to them that are innocent in nature coming from me but sound mischievous in nature if they were to come from anyone else. They need to not judge me on the basis of how an adult thinks, feels, wishes, desires, and needs things, but on the basis of how a child thinks, feels, wishes, desires, and needs things and have those childlike needs met in childlike ways.

They need to be willing to forgive me for anything that offends them and be wiling to go on as usual as if nothing ever happened.

They need to be able to show me this kind of forgiveness and still treat me with the exact same comfort and compassion they always did.

I need people to picture me in the eyes of a child and see me in the eyes of a child.

They need to treat me with the same continual pampering and reassuring words as they would a child.

Brian Evans
132

And, they need to always pull through with me in meeting all my comfort needs no matter what I say or do that may offend them.

If they are willing to do this for me and go on like they always have treating me with the same comfort and compassion they always have with no bias and no change in the way they are with me and everything always be the same then we have it made.

It is really important I receive this kind of affection and attention and is greatly needed on my end. I need to be able to receive hugs from all my doctors, nurses, and techs, and church members, and neighbors, and other friends I have made in public.

I have always required a lot of affection and attention.

Nurses need to have a deep understanding for who I am, how I think, and what is really going on in my mind. They need to understand just how childlike it is when I do say things that sound strange. This is what I need to feel I can go on.

Without this I will lose my will to live and I really need you to do this for me and be this accepting of me because this is really what I need from you.

I need a team of doctors and nurses and specialists and techs and hospital staff that understand all this and I'm hoping I've found all that now.

Have you guys ever seen the guy in the snow globe named Douglas that a girl in the real world tried to snatch away in the movie, "Snowglobe"?

That's the one that liked ice skating in the movie. He didn't get it about much of anything. He really didn't care for football either.

And he was the one who had a blonde girlfriend he hung out with in the globe. I'm a lot like him.

Brian Evans
133

What about the guy that plays Santa Claus in the movie "Snow"?

He's the one that constantly acts gullible and vulnerable in the movie. I'm a lot like him too.

Have you ever seen Gilligan on Gilligan's Isle? I'm a lot like him too.

If I hadn't been normalized you would be able to see it in a minute.

My normalization has blinded you from seeing this.

Once you take the intelligent looking facade away from all the education I've had and look into the eyes of the real person you see someone who thinks and acts almost exactly like these people. You'll be amazed and your eyes will be opened to the truth.

When I am finally able to open up to people and they are able to open up to me they will begin to see this as others already have.

I was simply trained to look like something else by a bunch of opera trainers for that play I was in and then I was also drilled like crazy memorizing facts out of books since the day I got out of special Ed.

It took me forever to catch up with everyone else intellectually.

When I finally did, I could finally understand some things you understand from the perspective of a book but when asked to apply them in a performance setting, "performing tasks on a job", what would be called experiments in a Science class, "I was lost as a goose about it".

For example, I could learn Medical Terminology and Anatomy and Physiology very well from memorization, but Medical Laboratory Procedures and Biology were hard for me because the "how to know how" of performance in these classes doesn't make sense to me and I did horrible in them.

As a result, I go work at a job, yes, and have a lot of knowledge, but where is my "know how" to run any equipment?

Where is my "know how" to figure out how to "perform any of the tasks on the job" which would be considered "experiments" in the classroom and not assignments?

Even in the 8th grade when I went into all regular classes after being in Special Ed the year before Anatomy and Physiology was the only class I made a B in. I made Cs in everything else.

The following semester when I took Physics, Chemistry, and Oceanography, those were also Cs.

This was not about a talent in Science.

This was about a talent in Anatomy and Physiology.

I was just good at that particular class and nothing else, not English, not History, not anything else.

I'm like one of these fact machines with a few talents that can't do anything else right.

If it's not in a book or one of my talents I'm lost.

I'm terrible at problem solving – knowing what to do in emergency situations.

When something comes up where I have to figure out what to do in an emergency situation I'm totally clueless.

I don't have a clue about what to do to take care of that emergency.

That's where the elevator does not hit the top floor in my head.

That's also why I cannot hold down a job because the "performance" area of my brain is shot, regardless of what I can do "academically".

Even most of the academics I took didn't turn out that great.
I would do well in Grammar and terrible at English Literature for example.

In High School Biology I would literally make As on the assignments and Fs on the experiments.

The book work made sense, the experiments did not.

That's the way my brain works.

I can know something is supposed to be a certain way but not be able to figure out how to perform it because I'm clueless.

Most of the classes I finally made As and Bs in were related to whatever my Major was at the time.

These were not in Music either.

Most of my music classes were also Cs except for Voice and Piano.

In both Music Theory and Intermediate Algebra I made 5 As, 5 Bs, 5 Cs, 5 Ds, and 5 Fs for approximately ever 25 assignments I turned in.

How's that for a jagged intelligence?

The logic involved in both of these classes is similar to each other but Music Theory is a little plainer than Algebra.

Brian Evans
136

It was my Medical Assisting classes, Medical Terminology Classes, Medical Transcription Classes, and Business classes I made most of my As and Bs in.

For some reason, I may be terrible in lab classes, but when it comes to book knowledge and file clerk skills in that area, that's where I've got the knack at.

I made Bs in History and Government in College unlike High School, but most of my other academics were actually Cs.

Most of my grades in High School were Cs too and I hated it.

Intermediate Algebra, Medical Laboratory Procedures, and Computer Electronics in took in college were Ds.

Computer Business I wound up being a B, but it was just basic, Word Perfect 5.1, Database3, Dos, Lotus.

I had some trouble with Dos and Lotus but did really well with Word Perfect 5.1 and Database 3. That's how I made the B.

Can you see how my intelligence jags?

I'm not the incredible genius most people think I am.

So, most people that think "he looks smart to me" or "he looks normal to me" aren't getting the point because they only see the things I "can do" that everyone else can do.
They fail to see the many other things I "can't do that other people can do".

And in most instances, everyone else has to be bad at something for me to be good at it. If their good at it I'm bad at it.

Strange isn't it?

That's where the elevator does not hit the top floor in my head.

That is why I cannot hold down a job. This is because the "performance" area of my brain is shot, regardless of what the "academic" can do.

I can know something is supposed to be a certain way but not be able to figure out how to perform it because I'm clueless.

Strange isn't it?

Most jobs are also too fast for me. They are too physically draining for me to handle so I am unable to hold out because of it.

Socially and emotionally I always have been and always be like what I was like when I was in Special Ed. Please see to it that you meet these needs and accept me the way I am. Thank you.

You see, with all these fears of what you will think of all these things I'm telling you and the completely twisted view of what is really going on I feel I cannot be myself because I feel like I have to walk on egg shells.

I feel like I cannot tell nurses what these "male" doctors, nurses, techs, and "serious trended female" nurses did to me in the past they may consider graphic because I fear they will think I am telling inappropriate stories about naked people when I am actually telling the truth.

My experience with the college girls where they thought all these horrible thoughts about me in this way that were untrue based on my body language make me terrified to tell you what these other people did in fear you will say, "We're sure not going to give you ladies now. Look what you are saying about these "so called" serious trended females. Were they really the serious trended females or did you just want us to think they were? They weren't the chipper ones, were they? Is there some reason you are asking for chipper people?" when the chipper acting female nurses were always the ones to show me the motherly compassion I need.

I fear you will keep "chipper acting female nurses" away from me based on false assumptions about how you think I think based on what a bunch of weirdo girls thought in college of me based on body language I was taught to have for some stupid play. I fear I will not get my needs met and will be treated roughly.

I am uncomfortable with men and serious trended women and need the comfort and compassion of motherly acting "chipper acting, cheery female nurses".

They are the only ones I am comfortable with and they are the ones I need. I always have and always will.

I have the mind of a child and I can't let your misconceptions of my childlike thoughts I have that you base on what normal people think that you judge me for stop you from giving me what I am asking for and what I need.

If you ever refrain from giving me what I need based on these false assumptions I will walk out on you and you will never see my face again even if I have an emergency.

It has to be chipper acting, cheery female nurses only.

I have to be able to be my Special Ed self with my childlike ways and have my childlike needs met.

Remember, one of your books says you are supposed to let your patient regress and act in childlike ways and have his childlike needs met.

This is what I want and this is what I need. I will not have it any other way.

It has to be "chipper acting, cheery female nurses" only.

I need "hugs" from all my nurses by letting me press my right ear on your cheek. I've needed this since infancy and have always had this need and it traumatizes me not to be able to do this with you. I am this way with everyone that I like.

I need one chipper acting female nurse to rub my head to calm me down and hold my hand through IVs, Blood tests, shots, biopsies, tube insertions, or anything else sharp while another chipper acting, cheery female nurse does the stick.

I need lots of affection and attention from all of them and be treated like I'm their own little boy.

I need to be able to look up to them like they are mommies and receive motherly compassionate care from all of them.

You do this and we're set.

You don't and there's no deal and I will be leaving. That's just the way it is. I cannot have it any other way and will not have it any other way.

Please do not refuse to meet my needs based on false assumptions from my past experiences.

Please do not refuse to meet my needs or refuse to give me who I ask for based on your misconception of anything I say, do, or ask from the mind of a child because you want to base it on what an adult would think if they asked for the same things.
I do not think like you and I am not wired like you.

I need different odd things from people for reasons that are totally innocent from the mind of a child who needs people.

I need them to see me for whom I am and meet all my special needs because that's what I am.

Brian Evans
140

I am autistic and I am a special needs person whether I appear that way to you or not.

If I had not been taken out of Special Ed and been normalized to the point you can't tell I have a problem without first getting around me a few months then I wouldn't have this problem. You would have no problem seeing the light.

Because this happened, it blinds you to the truth of what really is and always has been my true emotions of an ex Special Ed person with childlike thoughts and childlike needs.

To calm my anxiety over my fears of what people will think of me and how they will react to me and whether they will still meet my needs or not, the best thing they can do to resolve these fears is for everyone involved to say, "We know what your fears are and what we will think of you and you have nothing to fear because we believe you and we will meet all your needs as you asked us to." You do this and you will relieve a big burden off my chest and free me of my fears.

But, to keep me unafraid, you have to keep this promise and meet all my needs I ask you to meet every time and if I ever fear I've offended you reassure me immediately that everything is okay and you're alright.

If you reassure me immediately the minute you sense I fear you will think a certain bad thing about me or fear you will take offense to something and let me know immediately that everything is okay and your alright and I have done nothing to offend you, this will take a big weight off my chest.

You do these two things and continue to meet my needs as I ask you to, all of them, and I will gain confidence in your care dramatically after you've proved you'll really pull through for me with all of it. Then, we'll be set.

As far as the comfort measures go with the hugs, head rubs and hand holds through needle sticks and chipper acting cheery female nurses only who will give me lots of motherly love and affection I have to be able to have this because these are extremely detrimental needs to me.

If you don't do these particular things, the hugs, and the head rubs and hand holds through IV sticks, blood tests, shots, biopsies, and other sharp needle sticks I won't be sticking around, even if I am having an emergency.

If you don't believe me, ask my doctor.

She sent me to have a tetanus shot some place after I got a really bad bite from a Pit Bull Dog and they refused to give me the girls I wanted, refused to rub my head to calm me down and hold my hand, and refused to give me the shot in the hip. They insisted they were doing it in the arm. And, I wasn't sure they were going to give me hugs, either. When they did, I refused to take the shot and left.

My doctor had to call around until she found someone that would do all this for me and when she finally did they did really well for me and gave me hugs, chipper female nurses, rubbed my head to calm me down and held my hand, and gave me the shot in the hip.

If you do not do it my way, I will not be sticking around.
My needs are my needs and that's what I need.

If I ever go to the Emergency Room and they do not give me chipper acting female nurses and try to make me go with serious acting female nurses I will not be sticking around.

Male doctors and male nurses and techs and serious trended female nurses tortured me as a child.

The serious trended female nurses continued to torture me into adulthood.

Brian Evans
142

The Emergency Room has to do all this for me too, or I will not be sticking around for them either, even if I am having an emergency.

I seriously fear if I ever got a "serious trended" female nurse again if I refused to do an IV for them because I'm afraid of them they might actually try to take me by force and ram their IVs in me when they stick me with them.

I'm literally afraid of being tackled by them and thrown on a bed and pinned down to make me do whatever they ask. I'm even afraid of being forcibly stripped by them if I refuse to change into a hospital gown for them because I am afraid of them.

This would be the kind of nurses that act like the wicked witch of the west. I wanted to clarify that.

I am also terrified of all the male nurses doing this.

This is what they did to me at the military hospital and the institution.

I kind of doubt this happens where I am going now, but there are a couple of places I've been where the nurses really were forceful and I think someone like them might do this.

That place I went three years ago, there were three "serious trended" female nurses I almost got that didn't understand me at all.

They acted like they had every intention of forcing my every move if I went to them.

They never said they were going to, but they acted so mysterious about where I was supposed to go on the day of my procedure and were so straight-faced about everything, when they finally said "You'll be coming to us!" in a creepy tone of voice, I thought they were acting suspicious.

Anyone that's ever acted this way before toward me in the past has done this as a warning to let me know, "Watch out! If you come to us, you're going to get pounced! We're waiting for you, so be ready! We're about to give you the time of your life because we're your worst nightmare!"

What's funny is, the day I did go for my procedure there, the nurse I got let me know that my fears of what these people would do to me was not in vain. She let me know I was lucky I got her bunch.

The only problem is, her bunch started out nice, but when I was unable to make it through two IV stick attempts they got a "serious trended" female substitute IV sticker to do the stick and they swung it at me in the upper left arm like it was a shot and jabbed me good with it.

When I screamed and pulled my arm away, the same nurse that clarified how terrible these other nurses would act toward me yelled at me and said, "That's not allowed!" I said, "I can't help it! It hurt!" She was very mean about it.

I'm not going to refuse to cooperate with a "chipper acting cheery female nurse" as long as they meet my list of needs for hugs and comfort.

If they ask me to change into a gown for them for an examination or a procedure I will be more than happy to do so.

Just make sure to "never" give me a "male nurse" or a "serious trended female nurse" and we'll be okay.

It was the "male doctors", "male nurses" and "male" techs and "serious trended female nurses" that did this to me.

Their attitude is, "You're my property and you will do what I say".

They have always been very forceful with me and demanding and controlling.

Brian Evans
144

The chipper female nurses never did this to me.

They were nice to me if they ever got me and understood me and comforted me the way I needed to be comforted.

They were much nicer to me and much more compassionate than these other two types of nurses. It has to be chipper acting, cheery female nurses and techs only or there is no deal.

They are the ones I am comfortable with and they are the ones I need, not these other kinds of nurses.

Only the chipper acting, cheery female nurses will do.

And as far as Paramedics are concerned, if anyone ever calls you to come after me with an ambulance because I've had an accident, or I've passed out, am incredibly ill, or had chest pains and may or may not have had a heart attack or near heart attack, whatever it may be, "Never send any "male" paramedics to come get me!"
If something like this happens you send female paramedics.
I saw a man passed out at McDonald's in Branson last month and when the Paramedics came they sent three men to take care of him. When I saw this I panicked in my mind unknown to them thinking, "Don't ever give me a male! Never send me a male paramedic! They have to be female paramedics that are chipper that understand my comfort needs or I'm not going with them!"

I wasn't even the one being seen but the thought so pained me in my mind, I feared they'd automatically send me men if this happened to me, and I still say now, "Never send me a male paramedic, ever!"

Don't ever send me "serious trended female" paramedics either. It has to be "Chipper acting, cheery female paramedics, and techs, and nurses". No one else will do. If you send me "male" paramedics or "serious trended" female paramedics to me "I will not go with you". Never do this if you want me to cooperate with you.

Brian Evans
145

And you concerned callers, if you don't know if they know this information, you need to tell them to send Chipper acting, cheery female paramedics to come to my rescue or see if you can get a hold of my wife to see if she can take me herself. If she is unable to take me herself, this is who you need to have them send. No one else will do, no matter what the emergency is.

If you Paramedics want me to cooperate with you, as with all the other departments in the hospital and all the doctor office and hospital nurses and techs, they have to be "Chipper acting, cheery female nurses, techs, and paramedics "only". They have to "rub my head to calm me down and hold my hand through an IV stick". They all "have to give me hugs and let me give them hugs."

They have to let me put on Lidocaine/Prilocaine 2.5% cream on the site of the stick, preferably all over the arms and hands in case you fish around to see where you want to stick me at one hour before the stick. If you don't have that much time, at least put it on thick and wait to start in 15 minutes.

You "cannot put catheters or tubes in me awake, urinary or heart, or stomach". You have to "put me completely to sleep for "all" invasive procedures".
Even if you insist on doing the IV first, I need you to knock me out with the gas.

And, if you are willing to do so, please give me the gas for just long enough to make me feel numb and tingly and maybe somewhat woozy and then stick the IV needle in me. The inpatient ward you send me to has to follow these exact same procedures.

Not doing so will freak me out and I will walk out on you if you refuse to give me "Chipper acting, cheery female nurses only" and/or refuse to meet my childlike needs for comfort and hugs and/or refuse to rub my head to calm me down and hold my hand through an IV stick, Blood Test, or Shot.

Brian Evans
146

If you refuse to do any of these things, there is "no deal" on my end and you will not be able to keep me around to work on me because I will walk right out on you and leave, emergency or not.

I did this with the dog bite thing, and I will do this with everything else as well. Meet my needs or I'm out of there.

I know you are probably thinking in your mind that not all "serious trended female nurses" are like this.

I know there are a few "serious trended female nurses" out there that would never do this that just have a boring personality, but most of them would do something like this.

I know some of you are probably thinking, "I'll just make sure to give you one I know is going to be nice. They're just boring, but they won't hurt you." I still want a chipper acting one instead.

There have been a couple of instances where a doctor's office or hospital gave me one of these kind of "serious trended" female nurses which are one of the rare ones that are actually not mean after normally giving me the "chipper ones" they usually give me.

I think they thought, "Well, I know this nurse is "serious trended nurse", but they won't do anything to harm him. They're not like that."

I know, in these particular instances you were right if that's what you were thinking, but these particular nurses are not what I need even if they are not mean in nature.

Please understand. I don't mean to hurt these other nurses' feelings that just have a boring personality that mean no harm to me, but I feel more comfortable with the "chipper acting, cheery female nurses" and these other nurses are just not what I need.

I need the "cheery acting ones" to be the ones to help me and I have dependency needs that are childlike in nature.

Brian Evans
147

These "chipper acting cheery female nurses" are the best at meeting these needs for me and they are the ones I am comfortable with.

Even if a "serious trended female nurse" promises me they won't do this to me I will not cooperate with them, because I have to have the motherly love and comfort of all "chipper acting, cheery female nurses" and "chipper acting female techs."

Please, try to understand, and make sure you always give me "Chipper acting, cheery female" nurses and techs only. Thank you.

If the Emergency Room ever gives me male nurses instead of female nurses I will not be sticking around.

If they refuse to give me hugs in the Emergency Room, I will not be sticking around either.

If the Emergency Room refuses to give me chipper acting female nurses to rub my head to calm me down and hold my hand through an IV, blood test, or shot I will not be sticking around.
If I get the nurses I do want in the Emergency Room and they themselves refuse to rub my head to calm me down and hold my hand through needle sticks or give me hugs I will not be sticking around either.

I have to have "Chipper acting, cheery female nurses only" (these are female nurses with upbeat, cheerful personalities like people you would see on a Disney kid movie that perk you up and cheer you up). They all have to give me hugs, rub my head to calm me down and hold my hand through all IVs, blood tests, shots, biopsies, or other sharp needle sticks. They need to let me apply 2.5% Lidocaine/Prilocaine 1 hour before the stick. And I have to be put completely to sleep for all invasive procedures. No males or serious trended females can be present.

This also goes for Radiology techs, Anesthesiologists, Imaging Specialists, Rehabilitation staff, everybody, "chipper acting cheery female nurses" only with the same list of needs.

The same goes for Pre-Op, Radiology, Nuclear Medicine Imaging Services, Surgery, Colonoscopy and EGD, CCU, ICU, Cystoscopy, Rehabilitation Services, Pulmonology Services, Respiratory Care, In-Patient Care, Cardiac Cath Labs, Cardiology Surgery, Cardiology Testing Departments, or any other department of anyone's hospital anywhere.

The same also goes for Minor Emergency Clinics.

The same also goes for any doctor's office anywhere everywhere.

If my list of needs is not met, I will not be sticking around no matter who you are or where you are. So, please see to it that you meet my list of needs.

I also have a special request for my family doctor. If I ever have to go into the hospital for anything as an inpatient, can you come and visit me?

I really want to be able to see you if this happens. It would really mean a lot to me. Thanks.

I also want you to see something. When you see me, do you see this thing these opera people created that no one ever understood or do you see a special needs person from special Ed?

I was hoping you saw the second thing, because the first one is not the real me. It doesn't mean I don't have any talents. What I'm saying is that the whole problem was these girls were basing my personality on what these people made me look like and not based on who I am as an individual. What I was made to look like blinded these people from seeing the true me because of some weird body language I was taught to have that didn't even fit me.

Brian Evans
149

I think you already see the real me but I want to be sure you see the real me.

What the normal world sees since I got out of Special Ed is based on what they think Joe Blow down the street thinks when he says or asks or does the things he says or does or asks.

What the Special Ed world sees is this sweet little boy with special needs that thinks like a kid when he says the strange things he says or asks the strange questions he asks. They don't judge me based on how Joe Blow down the street thinks. They are judging me by how other Special Ed people think. If you judge me by how the every day person thinks every time I say something to you or ask you something or do something that looks strange you will be incorrect about how I am thinking about things almost every time. Their reasons for saying, asking and doing the things I say, ask and do are not the same as the reasons I say, ask, and do the things I say, ask, and do.

 If you think I said, asked, or did something because I thought what they thought or had their motives about something you will nearly always be incorrect, especially if the everyday person's motives for the same thing are bad. I'm not wired like everyday people. Special Ed people have different reasons for making the same statements and asking the same questions, kind of like the paint example I gave, a normal kid might want to vandalize a room if they ask for paint, but the special Ed kid just wants to paint a picture on a canvas. People have been punishing me all these years for things that aren't even the truth because they are basing it on the fact that, "Hey, he asked for paint. He must want to vandalize the room, because that normal kid over there wanted to vandalize the room when they asked me for paint." I'm not them. I know you think, "Well, that's just paint", but even some of the things I say that you might consider too personal or inappropriate in nature, may only be that way if one of them asked you the same thing. A special Ed person could say the same thing and just be cute and not mean anything bad at all by the same thing. A 5 year old for sure would.

Brian Evans

If a Special Ed person asked you to come visit them at the hospital it would be because they are needy people and you would be like another mommy to them. The same would for sure be the case for a 5 year old.

I just want you to see me as a child and treat me as a child and continue to comfort me and console me in the way you always have. I hope you don't mind because you're like a mother figure to me and I need to be able to have something like this. I just thought it would be nice if this were to happen if you could come up there and say, "Hey buddy. I heard you were in here. Are you okay? They said you were doing this way right now. I thought I'd come to see you to see how you were doing." and give me a hug and help comfort me. You would only have to step in for a few minutes. But, if you don't want bothered with it, don't worry about it. Just make sure they do this for me.

When I act all scared to ask you something like this it doesn't mean I'm guilty of anything wrong it just means that I am scared you will think I have something to be guilty about for asking this sort of question because you don't understand my need for this to happen and how important it is that my request be met.

I also tend to get scared when I struggle to tell you something I am too shy to ask you and fear you will show me your wrath if I say the wrong thing because you might interpret it differently from how I meant it. So, please keep this in mind when I do this. It doesn't mean I'm guilty of something bad. It just means I am struggling to tell you something because of fear of how you will take something or shyness I have about a subject I am asking you about, one of the two.

After being all scared my family doctor would misjudge me for asking her to visit me at the hospital if I was ever an inpatient for two or three days, I went to her office today and said, "You're going to think this sounds crazy, but, if I'm ever in the hospital for 2 or 3 days as an inpatient will you come visit me? I hope you don't mind."

Brian Evans
151

She said, "You think this is going to sound crazy. Of course, I will if you're in there." This made me feel a lot better. I thought she'd think I'd lost it but she didn't. I also feared she wouldn't actually have her daughter rub my head to calm me down and hold my hand through a blood test a 3rd time.

I was incredibly nervous and she could tell. She said, "Are you anxious? You don't have to be so anxious. Everything's going to be okay. We're going to do the same thing the same way we always do every time and my daughter is going to comfort you through the blood test every time the same way she always has. So, don't be worried okay. We're going to do this the same way every time."

That was an incredible relief and I felt a whole lot better.

I found this about comfort and compassion in Giving Emergency Care Competently about a burn victim I'd like to share with you.

"Granted, emergency care for a severely burned patient like Karen can be hectic. But don't forget she's a person who needs your strong emotional support. Burn patients experience excruciating mental stress from the shock of the accident, the pain, the chaos, and the rush to the hospital. Karen probably fears scarring and disfigurement. She needs you to be genuinely concerned for her welfare, and so does her anxious family. Tell her your name and call her by hers so she can feel the comfort of contact with another human being. Orient her to her surroundings and prepare her, as well as you can, for what she can expect."

> Giving Emergency Care Competently, Nursing Skillbook, page 153&154, Intermed Communications, Inc., 1979

I also found this long account about how nurses are supposed to comfort patients treated in the ICU unit.

I have always been afraid I would be treated impersonally if I ever went to someone's Intensive Care Unit (ICU) and I was amazed to find the following quote.

"Although the ICU, by nature, doesn't allow privacy or dignity, do what you can to make the patient feel less like an object. Don't talk about him at his bedside, unless he is included in these conferences. Handle his personal belongings with extra care – these are the only things in the ICU he can call his own, so they take on special meaning for him. Taking the time to stop and talk, or even to just be near the patient is extremely important."

"Touching" the patient's hand gently as you ask questions can help show him that you care. Don't forget to introduce yourself before you touch a patient and talk to him about the care as you give it, even if he's comatose or doesn't seem to respond. We've all probably had the experience of caring for a comatose patient, even of talking about him at his bedside, as if he didn't exist, only to have him tell us later exactly what had gone on around him. Try not to fall into this trap. Mr. Russell is not the "pneumonia on the ventilator" or a series of chest x-rays or blood-gas results. The complicated ICU gadgetry can distract you, but resist the temptation of thinking of patients and treating them as objects connected to this machinery. The best ICU nurse sees her patient first, the patient's condition second, and the equipment last. If the patient can't talk but can communicate, give him a magic slate, an alphabet board, or a clipboard, paper, and pencil, and encourage him to use it. If possible, try phrasing questions to allow for a simple yes or no answer. Use every opportunity to observe the patient's mental status, as well as his physical condition."

"If a patient seems depressed try to get him to think of the future rather than the not-very-pleasant present. Tell him when his family or friends call with a message and keep him aware of news and sports events- anything to get his mind off his illness. If a patient acts too independent, he's probably frightened of the helplessness he feels. Try to include him in decision making and to avoid restraining him when possible. Another patient may become totally dependent during illness and may look to an authority figure (like you) to solve all his problems." You may have to discourage this behavior once the patient's condition improves, but "it may be helpful to let him depend on you until then."

Brian Evans
153

Nursing the Critically Ill Patient, pages 30&32, Nursing
Skillbook, Intermed Communications, Inc., 1979

I don't care about sports so that wouldn't work with me.

I'm actually the one that would become totally dependent on you
and I'm technically already totally dependent on you due to my
disability of Autism.

"Also try to be aware of how the patient interacts with family
members. Remember, not all visits are beneficial, and destructive
relationships can add to the patient's stress. If certain visitors seem
to upset your patient, try to find out why and work with other
members of the family to remedy the situation."

Nursing the Critically Ill Patient, pages 30&32, Nursing
Skillbook, Intermed Communications, Inc., 1979

I have always been a dependent person and have always been
dependent on others with dependency needs and need to be able to
be dependant on my nurse when I am in the hospital setting.

"To care for any patient with colorectal cancer, you must be three
people in one: the efficient nurse who gives fine in-hospital care,
the "compassionate" nurse who gives "emotional support", and the
instructive nurse who teaches the patient home care."

Helping Care Patient's Efficiently, Nurseskillbook, page
95, Intermed, Inc. 1977

"Before surgery, your goals include preparing the child for surgery
– first psychologically by telling him what to expect before,
during, and after surgery – without intensifying his anxiety. Then
you physically prepare him, while offering emotional support and
reassurance. And you must prepare his parents to support and
reassure him throughout this terrifying crisis. Children like David
are usually admitted 2 to 5 days before surgery to prepare them
emotionally and physically, and to complete routine studies.

Many hospitals give them and their parents a tour of the unit and information about the surgery. Even after such orientation, you'll find most children and their parents in a highly anxious state. Parents like David's have known for a long time that surgery was inevitable for his survival. They've surely tried to prepare themselves and their child for this frightening event. Still they can't help feeling overwhelmed by their fear of what may happen."

"Parents with any unresolved guilt or inability to accept the child's defect will have much difficulty. They'll show it by being very demanding – asking many questions…looking for frequent attention and seemingly insignificant thins and reasons…and even acting hostile. You need to realize this is not directed at you personally. Try to spend time with them. Allow them to express their anxiety, guilt, and frustrations. Doing so will help the child indirectly; his anxiety will, to some extent mirror theirs. Also remember the many sources of the child's anxiety. Many children David's age view hospitalization and painful procedures as punishment for misbehavior or bad thoughts. They are still egocentric. David's anxiety may be rooted in fear of: separation from his parents, loss of parental love, punishment or physical harm. He may fear needles, cuts, and foreign objects on his body. He may have a heightened awareness of his body, an exaggerated concern for privacy, and may be overly modest – refuse hospital gowns, "forget" to save urine specimens, shun rectal temperatures, and deny constipation. Older school-age children may fear abandonment, body mutilation, and death. But don't go by chronological age alone. It may be misleading. Regression is a normal and expected defense mechanism at any age: It allows the threatened person to fall back on earlier coping mechanisms. But it is frightening. The child who regresses realizes his immature inclinations, but cannot accept or control his response."

> Combatting Cardiovascular Diseases Skillfully, Nursing Skillbook, pages 33 &34, Intermed Communications Inc., 1978

It helps me to get a tour of the procedure room and meet all the nurses first to see what they are like the day before the procedure.

If I do I know who to ask for based on who I'm comfortable with. I need to know whether they are chipper acting, cheery female nurses in my view or not. This way I can see which nurses are chipper and which ones are not. I need to know whether they will be willing to meet my needs. And, I'll be able to see for myself what they are willing to do for me. All this has to be established in the beginning. My needs have to be met or I cannot go through with the procedure. They have to all be chipper acting, cheery female nurses and techs that act like someone of a Disney kid movie. These chipper nurses all have to give me hugs and be willing to give me hugs when I go in for the procedure before, during and after the procedure. These chipper nurses also need to be willing to rub my head to calm me down and hold my hand through IVs, Blood tests, Shots, Biopsies, tube insertions, blades, scalpels, or any other sharp needle sticks. They also need to knock me completely out for every invasive procedure including "cardiac catherization" or any other invasive procedure.

This book actually talks about them talking to the patient while they do it and having them do different things for them. This will not work for me.

I have to be completely asleep and completely numb.

I cannot have any idea what you are doing to me when you perform you "cardiac catherization" procedure on me, or a "Transesophageal Echocardiogram" on me, or any other invasive procedure on me. This is true even if it is just urinary catheters or stomach tubes, or the like. I have to be put to sleep for all this.

Plus, it is not good enough to just give me a tour and let me meet all the nursing staff and make me familiar with the equipment and what will happen to me. That helps, but the only way to get me through a procedure is to give me the chipper acting female nurses and techs I am asking for only, give me hugs, and rub my head to calm me down and hold my hand through all needle sticks. You do that and we have it made. You don't and I won't be coming your way.

Brian Evans
156

If you trick me and tell me you won't after you promised you would, I will literally walk out of the room and go home if I have the least notion that you will not meet my needs on my list I am asking you to meet.

You refuse to meet any of my needs and there's no deal. Either meet my list of needs or forget the whole thing.

That will also be the case even if I have an emergency.

You should be willing to "touch" me in addition to just talking to me. Even adult patients are supposed to be allowed to regress to childlike ways and be able to have their childlike needs met. My needs are my needs and this is what I need. I will not accept impersonal care from anyone.

"Touch is a primal need, as necessary as food, growth or shelter. Think of "touch" as a nutrient transmitted through the skin and "skin hunger" as a form of malnutrition that has reached epidemic proportions in the United States, especially among older persons." Older adults need touch as much or more than any other age group. Simple touch helps older adult clients feel more connected to and accepted by those around them and to their environment."
Fundamentals of Nursing, 7th Edition, Potter and Perry, Mosby Elsevier, 2009, page 784

"In illness it should be expected that patients will regress to levels of behavior that are not as mature as those which they assume when well. They need to be allowed sufficient and appropriate regression and dependence in others. Ill persons have a strong 'need' for security, 'warm', friendly interactions and familiar settings promote feelings of security." In their search for security patients often hope to find in nurses the reassuring qualities of sympathy, tenderness, understanding, and gentleness tempered with firmness. The careful reader will observe that these are qualities often attributed in the "ideal mother figure."
Basic Nursing: A Psychophysiologic Approach, Sorenson Luckmann, W.B. Saunders Company, 1979, page 152

"Patients express frustration with the impersonal and diffuse care received in many large institutional settings. The nurse's focus should be on ensuring the preservation of personalism and continuity of care."

> Comprehensive Rehabilitation Nursing, Nancy Martin, Nancy B. Holt, Dorothy Hicks, McGraw Hill Book Company, 1981, page 569

"To reinforce what I've already said about not needing an elaborate conversation with the patient, I suggest you try to remember a time when you yourself were really down and just prayed for someone who would understand. Chances are, you weren't looking for a lot of talk, but for someone who simply would listen and not be afraid to "touch" you." If you can remember such a time, and most of us can, then you will know that you need to leave your "armor of professionalism" outside the door. Patients often feel repulsive, freaky, and unclean. "Touching" them, "putting a hand on their hand" or on the "nape of their neck" can mean so much, can make it a truly caring encounter. If only we could be honest, both admit our fears and "touch" one another. If you really care, would you lose so much of your valuable professionalism if you cried with me? Just person to person? Then, it might not be hard to die…in a hospital…with friends close by."

> Dealing with Death and Dying, page 32, Nurseskillbook, Intermed Inc., 1980

Actually, this would make it easier to live for me, but only after continuously being this way with me when in a period of stress or grief. I am already a very "touchy feely" person in the first place and need this kind of thing on a continual basis anyway, but I need it all the more during stress or grief, to a very great extent.

"The emphasis on comfort and the role it plays in health care has changed in the last 10 decades. From 1900 to 1929, comfort was the central focus and moral imperative of nursing: from 1930 to 1959, comfort was considered a strategy for achieving fundamental requirements of nursing care: and from 1960 to 1980, comfort fell out of favor, to become only a minor aspect of nursing, and was significant only to people who received no medical treatment."

> Chia-Chia, Lin, PhD, School of Nursing, Taiwan
> Comfort: A Value Forgotten in Nursing-Lin, Chia-Chia
> PhD, RN, Cancer, Nursing: November/December 2010-
> Volume 33, Issue 6-pp409-410

"During the last 3 decades, comfort has been relegated to end-of-life care where it is equated with the simplest aspects of care, which could be just as easily provided by nonprofessional caregivers."

> Chia-Chia, Lin, PhD, School of Nursing, Taiwan
> Comfort: A Value Forgotten in Nursing-Lin, Chia-Chia
> PhD, RN, Cancer, Nursing: November/December 2010-
> Volume 33, Issue 6-pp409-410

"Today, as always, comfort remains a substantive need throughout our oncology nurses play an important role in promoting comfort through their lives. Comfort is not a novel idea and has been cited by prestigious and cancer patients. In conclusion, comfort should not be relegated to end-of-life care. There is a powerful need for an increase in translational research to promote comfort in every stage of patient care. When comfort is emphasized in nursing care and when promoting comfort becomes an important core value of nursing, I believe that nurses will gain more respect from their patients, the families of patients, and our colleagues in the field of medicine."

> Chia-Chia, Lin, PhD, School of Nursing, Taiwan
> Comfort: A Value Forgotten in Nursing-Lin, Chia-Chia
> PhD, RN, Cancer, Nursing: November/December 2010-
> Volume 33, Issue 6-pp409-410

Please remember this when you take care of me. Thanks.

Dear Nurses,

Please note my needs when you take care of me. I appear to be normal but I am actually autistic and have childlike needs. I need a lot of affection from cheery acting, chipper female nurses with motherly personalities who are caring and compassionate and willing to comfort me the way I ask them to comfort me. I have a sensory issue in my right ear that can only be relieved by putting my right ear on the cheek of the people I like, I call doing this a hug. So, I need to be able to do this with my nurses as well to bring me comfort, especially in medical situations, and I need to do it even worse when I'm scared. A cheery acting female nurse also needs to rub the top of my head and hold my hand to comfort me through an IV stick, blood test or shot, while another cheery acting female nurse does the stick. They also need to do this for me if I have a biopsy awake or have to be stuck with or cut with any other sharp instruments. It is really important I have these met. Those who have done this for me in the past did really well with me. I have a fear of needles and oversensitivity to pain. A shot and a blood test feel like being stuck with a steak knife. An IV feels like being stabbed with a butcher knife. A catheter feels like a sword being run through me. I need to be able to put Lidocaine/Prilocaine 2.5% cream on the site of the stick because of this. I need to be knocked out for all invasive procedures, as well as any catheter or tube insertions. I also need all the radiology techs and anesthesiologists and everybody that deals with me needs to be cheery, chipper acting females only and I need to be able to put my right ear on their cheek too because of my sensory issue. Male doctors, nurses, and techs tortured me as a child so I am scared of men. The serious trended female nurses also tortured me in childhood and adulthood so I am scared of them too. Please give me chipper acting, cheery female nurses to work with me only.

Your friend,

Brian Gene Evans

Dear Nurses,

For those of you who are unable to catch what all of my needs are on the letter you just saw who need to see them in list form, here is my list of needs again. Please meet all these needs on this list. Not doing so traumatizes me, so it's very important you meet these.

- Need All Chipper Acting, Cheerful Female Nurses Only
- No Male Nurses, Therapists, Techs, Radiologists, or Anesthesiologists
- No Serious Trended Female Nurses, Therapists, Techs, Radiologists, or Anesthesiologists
- Need Hugs from All My Nurses (A Hug to Me is Putting my Right Ear on Your Cheek)
- Need a Chipper Acting, Cheerful Female Nurse to Rub my Head to Calm me Down and Hold my Hand While Another Chipper Acting Female Nurse does the IV, Blood Test, or Shot
- They Also Need To Do This For Me If Any Biopsies are taken awake, or any Blades, Or Scalpels, or Other Sharp Instruments Are Used On Me Awake
- I Need to Be Able to Put on Lidocaine/Prilocaine 2.5% Cream on Site of Stick
  One Hour Before A Needle Stick of Any Kind
- Need to Be Knocked Out For Any Catheter Insertions or Tube Insertions
  (Heart or Urinary Catheter Insertions)
* Need to Be Able to Write Doctors/Nurses About Any Medical Conditions/Symptoms   I Have or Any Emotional Needs I Need Met
* Need All Medical Professionals Dealing With Me to Be Informed of the Needs
  On this List and Be Willing to Meet Them

You meet this list and we are good to go. I still need to hug everyone I see so don't just limit it to one or two people that specifically work with me.

Brian Evans
161

I need to be able to hug everybody I see when I go for a test in the Radiology Department for example, or the Pre-Op Department for example. Being able to do this helps me to be able to feel safe in my environment and comfortable with my nurses with the reassurance that anyone who does any other test on me in the same department will always be the same way with me as well as the ones that work with me, but do still only give me the chipper acting female nurses only to work with me because they are the nurses I am comfortable with. Plus, I have a sensory issue in my right ear that can only be relieved by being able to place my right ear on the cheek of all the people I like, including nurses. Not only that, but there are some tests that are so difficult for me to handle you may need extra assistance at times as well, so it is also better that everybody be prepared to give me a hug so I can feel at ease with everyone and know I will be taken care of in the way I need cared for with the comfort I need to receive from them in the way I need to receive it from them and not by what they decide but by how I tell them they need to comfort me, by giving me hugs, let me press my right ear on their cheek, and rub my head to calm me down and hold my hand through needle sticks. I need chipper acting cheery female nurses only to work with me.

The chipper acting cheery female nurses are the most compassionate people that do better at comforting me and making me feel at ease than anyone else. Male nurses and serious trended nurses tortured me as a child. Serious trended female nurses also tortured me as an adult. I need the chipper acting female nurses only to work with me that have cheery motherly personalities and comfort me the way I state I need comforted and I will be good to go. I am autistic and have childlike needs and need to be comforted in the way I ask to be comforted because this is the only thing that works for me. Please see to it that this is done for me, and we're set to go. Thank you.

Your friend,

Brian Gene Evans

Also available are:

"Big City Hospitals Don't Like Cowards" by Brian Gene Evans

"To Nurse Means to Nurture: The Need for Nurses to Comfort their Patients" by Brian Gene Evans

"To Nurse Means to Nurture Part Two: The Parent Role of Nurses of All Ages of Patients" by Brian Gene Evans

"Mainstreaming a Disabled Person into the Normal World is a Big Mistake" by Brian Gene Evans

"Compassion for Disabled Peers in College is Needed" by Brian Gene Evans

"What Language Therapy Really Entails" by Brian Gene Evans

"Autism Undiagnosed: What Happened?" by Bertha Marie Evans

"Autism Undiagnosed Part II: Will I Always Be an Outcast?" by Bertha Marie Evans

"Joys and Sorrows of Living with Adult Autism" (Autism Undiagnosed Part III) by Bertha Marie Evans

"Victory" by Bertha Marie Evans

"How to Have a Happy Marriage" by Bertha Marie Evans

If anybody has any questions about anything they read in this book please contact, my wife, Bertha Marie Evans at (870) 416-1030.